CW00347400

HOW TO
AVOID CANCER

For
MICHI and DANIELE,
my delightfully sensible daughters

HOW TO
AVOID CANCER
Dr Jan de Winter

JAVELIN BOOKS
POOLE · DORSET

First published in the UK 1985 by Javelin Books,
Link House, West Street, Poole, Dorset, BH15 1LL

Copyright © 1985 Dr Jan de Winter

Distributed in the United States by
Sterling Publishing Co., Inc.,
2 Park Avenue, New York, NY 10016

British Library Cataloguing in Publication Data

De Winter, Jan
  How to avoid cancer.
  1. Cancer—Prevention
  I. Title
  616.99′405   RC268

ISBN 0 7137 1593 6

All rights reserved. No part of this book may
be reproduced or transmitted in any form or by any
means, electronic or mechanical, including
photocopying, recording or any information
storage and retrieval system, without
permission in writing from the publisher.

This book is sold subject to the conditions that
it shall not, by way of trade or otherwise, be
lent, re-sold, hired out or otherwise circulated
without the publisher's prior consent in any form
of binding or cover other than that in which it
is published and without a similar condition
including this condition being imposed on
the subsequent purchaser.

Typeset by Colset Pte Ltd, Singapore.

Reproduced, printed and bound in Great Britain by
Hazell Watson & Viney Limited,
Member of the BPCC Group,
Aylesbury, Bucks

CONTENTS

HOW TO AVOID CANCER
Dr Jan de Winter

In Britain alone cancer, at present, claims the life of one person every three minutes; yet the tragic irony of this is that cancer can be shown to be avoidable in about half the people currently dying from it.

The more common forms of cancer — lungs, breast, bowel, uterus and throat — are often the results of years of self abuse and unhealthy living. Dr Jan de Winter maintains that obesity, heavy smoking and drinking, stress, easy sex and in particular excessive, over-rich food-intake are the root factors contributing to many of the unnecessary cancer deaths in recent time.

What is special about this book is that it reveals how to reduce the risks and thereby the likelihood of contracting cancer. Because of its prolonged and yet so treacherously silent induction-period, sometimes extending over twenty or more years, cancer can be arrested and the malignant process reversed at any stage early on, by exchanging unhealthy habits for a more sensible way of living, thereby making life more fully enjoyable for so much longer.

In this book Dr de Winter outlines his plan for a healthy life by controlling diet, weight, smoking and drinking and so making our bodies fitter and thus more capable of withstanding the onslaught of this terrible disease.

From 1950 to 1981 Dr Jan de Winter was Senior Consultant in charge of cancer treatment for the whole of Sussex at Brighton's Royal Sussex County Hospital. During this time he earned an international reputation as a cancer specialist and he continues now to wage, single-handed, a constant campaign to prevent cancer by advancing public education in health.

In 1967 Dr de Winter brought into being, in Brighton, Copper Cliff, one of the United Kingdom's leading hospices for needy cancer sufferers. Dr de Winter is also the founder of Brighton's Whole Body Scanner Department, inaugurated in 1976, where he pioneered his revolutionary technique of pinpointing deep-seated cancer for subsequent precision-treatment, a method now used routinely in all cancer centres. In 1982 Dr de Winter founded his High Street Clinic for Cancer Prevention Advice in Brighton*, the first such clinic in all of Europe, where anyone, on an impulse, can just walk in and find out free of charge how to reduce the likelihood of contracting cancer.

*6, New Road; telephone 0273–727213.

Part One

CANCER AND ITS PREVENTION

1 THE NATURE OF CANCER AND ITS CAUSES

That Paolo Mantegazza's much-quoted century-old dictum, which says that 'Out of a Hundred Diseases, Fifty Are Caused by Our Own Faults, Forty by Our Carelessness', should still be valid in the enlightened 1980s is especially lamentable since the two most frequently lethal self-inflicted diseases are heart disease and cancer. Currently, cancer claims the life of one citizen every three minutes. This is because it affects one person in every four in the Western world and this it will continue to do until we alter our so-called civilised way of life.

Basically, the destructive process within us that we call cancer can originate in the body only because of the remarkable ability of living tissue to compensate for abuse, injury or damage by initiating an acceleration of cellular activity, thereby forming new tissue with which to repair the damage. Normally this is a highly orderly and strictly time-limited process.

However, when the factors causing the abuse, injury or damage, such as dietary excesses, addiction to cigarettes or over-consumption of alcohol, are repetitive, that is when they continue to operate both regularly day after day and indefinitely year after year, then the body's attempt at repair will eventually become disorderly and will escalate into unrestrained cellular activity ultimately culminating in uncontrolled growth: cancer.

It is entirely up to each individual to rid the body of the repetitively damaging factors and thereby avoid some forms of cancer altogether. All that is necessary is to become conversant with the predisposing damaging factors and, once this knowledge is acquired, to exercise the self-discipline necessary to translate this knowledge into practice by taking full charge of one's own body, making the maintenance of good health a strictly personal responsibility of the highest priority.

As the natural cancer death rate shows, this responsibility can be relinquished or delegated to others (such as doctors or the government) only at dire peril to one's own survival. This is the reason why, after heart failure, cancer leads the death league-table as second main cause of death, and why in 1981 cancer claimed the lives of over 146,970 victims in the United Kingdom, that is 12,000 every month or 400 every day or one cancer death every three minutes.

Why, of all the words in a doctor's vocabulary, is there none more frightening to patients than the verdict of 'cancer'? It is because the disease can be likened to an implacable enemy lurking deep inside each and every one of us, lying in wait, silent, invisible, malevolent, biding its time perhaps for twenty years or more, seemingly dormant but always poised and ready to pounce as soon as one's own usually impregnable body defences have been eroded, whittled away, worn down, mortally weakened and finally destroyed by years and years of careless, irresponsible, pleasure-related self-abuse.

It is not universally realised that it is as a result of human fallibility that the more common forms of preventable cancer arise and continue to claim year after year, inexorably, heartbreakingly and *so* unnecessarily the lives of thousands of unenlightened and therefore unsuspecting victims. To their bewildered question as to what it is that exacts this supreme penalty with such relentlessness and frequency the answer must always be: *the stubbornness of our own personal habits.*

Human nature being what it is, namely self-indulgent, pleasure-seeking and more often than not somewhat short-sighted, personal habits even when known to be harmful to health are rarely changed except under duress, that is, when they have started to cause troublesome ailments such as indigestion, high blood pressure, a duodenal ulcer, diabetes, gout etc. As long as these conditions are amenable to treatment they are reversible.

Cancer, which is also induced by personal habits, is *irreversible* on account of the treacherously long induction time. Induction time is the silent period between the first exposure to whatever it is in our personal habits that causes cancer and the actual visible appearance of the growth. This averages two to three decades before reaching its malignant invasive stage. During this time the disease is potentially arrestable and reversible by the body's own intrinsic physiological and immunological defence mechanisms, always provided that these mechanisms have not been weakened or damaged by years and years of dietary or other excesses.

Types of cancer

The outstanding property of a cancer cell is its loss of control over its own replication. As a result the rate of multiplication will no longer match the rate of routine cell-loss due to wear and tear; it will exceed it and this results in tumour formation.

Cancer cells that arise in the epithelium (the surface-lining of the skin and various other organs) are called carcinomas, whereas sarcomas develop in tissues supporting bone cells, blood vessels, fibrous connective tissue and muscle.

There is a heterogenous group of cancers comprising Hodgkins Disease, lymphosarcoma and leukaemia, the latter originating in the blood forming bone marrow cells, the former two in the lymphatic system. More than 90 per cent of human cancers are (epithelial) carcinomas and less than 10 per cent are sarcomas and leukaemias.

Childhood cancers (and those arising in animals) are usually leukaemias and sarcomas, whereas cancers occurring in adults are mostly carcinomas.

In all about 200 distinct varieties of cancers are recognised in man, but for the purpose of cancer prevention only the four more readily avoidable types of cancer, namely cancer of the breast, bowel, lung and skin, will be discussed.

Of these, skin cancer is most curable, whereas the other three forms, breast, bowel and lung cancer, together are responsible for over half of all cancer deaths. Depending on the organ of their origin, these four forms of cancer show a very wide range of behaviour.

In the skin, the epithelium can be subdivided into two distinct sections: the epidermis or top layer and the underlying dermis. The top layer is usually 5–10 cells deep and continually replaces itself by cell division in its deepest basal layer next to the dermis.

In addition to epithelial cells, the epidermis cells also contain pigment-cells, called melanocytes, which synthetise granules containing the dark brown pigment, melanin, which is incorporated into the maturing multi-plying basal cells; the function of these melanocytes is to protect the basal cells from ultraviolet light.

There are two common cancers of the skin and one less common one; the latter, however, is potentially much more deadly, because it originates in the skin-melanocytes; all three forms of skin cancer are frequently induced by excessive sunlight.

The first of these three skin cancers is the rodent ulcer or basal cell carcinoma which, as the name suggests, arises in the basal cell layer; it does not metastasize and is, therefore, eminently curable., Its name, cancer, is actually a misnomer, because of its benign behaviour and extreme cura-bility. It is easily recognisable because it forms an ulcer (skin defect) with rolled undermined edges and a small central crust, which keeps falling off and reforming. It slowly enlarges in all directions and if left untreated can reach an enormous size. Its site of predilection is the face.

The second skin tumour, the squamous carcinoma, which frequently resembles a peeled tomato, is, as the name implies, made up of squamous epithelium and can occasionally spread to the regional lymphnodes. It is also readily curable.

5

These two types of skin cancer are usually treated by radiotherapy, using superficially acting 'soft' X-rays; however, surgical excision is equally effective. With extensive lesions the results of surgery may be cosmetically less satisfactory.

Finally, the third skin cancer, the melanoma, arises in the skin's melanocytes. It has a notorious tendency to blood-borne spread and thus to distant metastases. The incidence of melanoma has been steadily increasing all over the world as a result of the greater exposure to the sun dictated by the current fashion to 'wear' a tan, that is to have a bronzed body. A melanoma necessitates radical surgical excision.

Melanomas almost invariably arise in pigmented moles, present for many years, sometimes since birth. When the colour of such a mole deepens, when it becomes larger and thicker and when there is some bleeding from the lesion (the cardinal triad of symptoms indicating an active lesion), the diagnosis of a melanoma can no longer be in doubt.

The person with a melanoma, surprisingly, is not the man or woman who has spent a lifetime in an outdoor occupation and who has a high, total lifetime-dose of natural sunlight. He or she is more at risk to develop one of the other two types of skin cancer — either a basal cell carcinoma or a squamous cell carcinoma. The patient with a melanoma is usually two to three decades younger and is most often an indoor office worker of higher socio-economic status. There usually is a correlation between a severe sunburn and development of melanoma in the following five years, suggesting that short episodes of intense burning sunlight-exposure are a risk factor, as is exposure of areas other than face and hands, particularly in people who do not tolerate ultraviolet light exposure well and easily freckle.

The beauty of a tanned body became fashionable in the 1940s; by the mid-1950s the epidemic of skin cancers began, mainly in people with a fair complexion who find it difficult to get tanned. These people should always apply a barrier sun-cream containing an ultraviolet light protection factor which screens the skin from the effects of the sun; additionally they should wear a hat and long-sleeved shirt or blouse, particularly on the beach or on the skiing slopes.

Cancer arising in the epithelium of the breast mostly forms a hard nodule, which is readily detectable in the soft tissue of the breast on self-examination. The diagnosis is established by a needle-biopsy during which a few cells from the nodule are aspirated for subsequent microscopic examination. Breast cancer is usually treated surgically. Until recently this meant routine amputation of the affected breast. Of late the patient may elect to have a more conservative operation instead, in the form of a local 'lumpectomy'. Depending on the involvement of axillary lymphnodes, postoperative radiotherapy may be advisable.

Breast cancer occurs most frequently in virgins and childless women.

The prognosis after surgery depends less on the treatment given than on the tumour's metastatic tendency. This is why the disease still kills about 14,000 women every year. In fact, true cure-rates have probably changed very little since 1950.

Lung cancer (annual death rate about 40,000) which arises predominantly in smokers, is virtually incurable; it occurs only very exceptionally in non-smokers. The Royal College of Physicians estimates that at least 100,000 deaths in the UK each year are caused by smoking-related diseases. The risk to health induced by smoking will be discussed in a separate chapter. Lung cancer is usually diagnosed by a combination of radiological findings on chest X-ray, and on bronchoscopy (during which the tumour is viewed through a periscope-type of instrument passed through mouth and throat right down to visualise the appropriate bronchus). The most significant clinical sign of lung cancer, apart from a chronic cough and dyspnoea (shortness of breath) on exertion, is the coughing up of a blood-stained sputum.

Bowel cancer claims at least 19,000 victims each year. Obese people, particularly those who tend to eat a lot of red meat and rich, fatty foods, are especially prone to contracting bowel cancer. The success of treatment, which invariably consists of surgical excision of the affected bowel section, depends on the advancement of the condition at operation, that is on the local extension of the disease, on involvement of regional lymphnodes and, of course, on the presence of distant spread to other organs, in particular to the liver.

The diagnosis of bowel cancer is made by means of an X-ray examination of the contrast-filled bowel (called a barium enema) and confirmed further by colonoscopy during which the tumour can be directly viewed through a pliable, i.e. fibre-optic, instrument that can be passed the whole length of the bowel right up to the tumour. The earliest sign of bowel cancer is the presence of occult blood, detectable on a chemical test of the stools in the laboratory.

What makes cancer such a fell disease is its own particular mode of spread. Similar to seeds of ordinary garden weeds that are carried by the wind or by water to other parts of the garden where, having been deposited, they start to grow again, so cancer cells are carried by the blood stream or lympth stream from the original site to other parts of the body where they may set up fresh secondary satellite growths. It is as a result of this Russian-roulette type of lethal yet unpredictable dissemination that cancer is so hazardous a disease.

By contrast, what is more predictable, because it is usually determined by the patient's personal habits, is the organ which is to undergo malignant change. For instance, cigarette smoking affects the lungs; pipe smoking usually attacks the lip or the tongue; too much alcohol affects the upper air and digestive passages; strong coffee can damage the pancreas; too much beer may injure the rectum; dietary excesses tend to attack the intestine and the breast; whereas obesity increases the risk of cancer of the body of the uterus, ovary, breast and gallbladder.

Cures

The outcome of treatment in each single case of cancer is uncertain because of the very nature of the disease, whose spread to other parts of the body is so notoriously unpredictable. There are three definitive forms of treatment — surgery, radiotherapy and chemotherapy — and in all three, when they were first introduced, the aim of treatment was palliation (alleviation of symptoms only).

Historically, surgery was the first form of 'curative' treatment; then as now, this method depended for success on the tumour being excisable and confined solely to the site of excision, a set of circumstances which is uncommon in cancer.

When radiotherapy was introduced, it was used chiefly as palliative treatment, but many tumours, particularly skin tumours, are now curable by radiotherapy when employed as the sole form of treatment.

Chemotherapy has developed only in the past fifteen to twenty years, and it has been possible to use the word cure of late in four types of malignant disease (acute lymphoblastic leukaemia in children, choriocarcinoma of pregnancy, Hodgkin's Disease and testicular tumours). In these conditions the offending cancer cells are found to be more sensitive to damage by the drugs than the normal cells — and therefore these diseased cells can be eradicated without permanent harm being caused to the healthy ones.

There is a fourth, newer, still experimental form of treatment, called immunotherapy. This method, not yet established, can be used only when the number of malignant cells is very small, i.e. it can be employed only as an aid to other forms of treatment.

It must be apparent from the preceding remarks that, however early a tumour is diagnosed and treated, there can be no guarantee of a cure, because no two cancers can be expected to respond in an identical fashion, for the simple reason that their individual characteristics, such as for instance their rate of cell division or their propensity to distant spread, vary as indeed does the host's immunological response and resistance to these invading cells. It therefore follows that a reliably effective cure for cancer will become possible only when we have acquired additional knowledge, in particular as regards the fundamental mechanics of cell growth, something that will take many more decades, if not centuries, to come about.

Let us take breast cancer as a concrete example to illustrate this point. The reason why treatment fails to 'cure' breast cancer in a high proportion of patients is simply that the malignant cells disseminate throughout the body when the primary growth is still small, and though local treatment by surgery and radiotherapy is effective there is no curative treatment for metastatic (spreading) disease, and it is metastatic disease which kills.

Long-term follow-up studies show that even in so-called 'early' disease 70 per cent of patients will sooner or later die of breast cancer, their death being related to their metastatic disease.

Chemotherapy in most solid tumours, using drugs or hormones, has failed to show any improvement in patient long-term survival. The only constant finding is that chemotherapy has toxic side-effects.

Prevention

As has already been stated, in about half of all patients who eventually die from it, cancer is a self-inflicted disease. Despite this now being public knowledge, imprudent dietary habits, addiction to cigarettes and habitual over-consumption of alcohol are still accepted by today's self-indulgent consumer society, aided and abetted by unscrupulously slanted and totally profit-motivated commercial advertising, as an integral part, if not undisputed highlight, of everyday life.

In a free democratic society, the prerogative to pursue one's own behaviour pattern and to choose one's personal life-style still remains a birthright which no-one so far has ventured to challenge. This automatic right to unrestricted freedom of choice of one's own way of life at an early age is tantamount, in the eyes of one dedicated by vocation to the care of the sick and the dying, to an official licence, or even more than that, to an open invitation to commit slow, insidious suicide in public. The price of this statutory carte-blanche for optional self-extinction is not only absolutely exorbitant in terms of unnecessary suffering for patients and their loving relatives; it is also unacceptably prohibitive in terms of needless loss of life, both from preventable cancer and from the other four killer diseases — liver cirrhosis, stroke, chronic bronchitis and heart failure.

It is important to assure the reader that the author is neither a puritanical health fanatic who expects everyone to emulate the hypochondriac who lived his life as an invalid so that he could die healthy; nor that he is a

9

sanctimonious scaremonger who wants to frighten everyone into submission. His sole aim is to turn today's tragedies to the reader's advantage by using them as lessons for tomorrow's better health so that fewer and fewer people will be willing so readily to accept the high personal health risks that are associated with many of today's pleasurable pursuits. It is only when society will have become conversant with cancer's prime causes that these will be readily recognised and can then be actively avoided.

This is the only practical way — and what an unpopular one it is — to make a major impact on today's risk of death from cancer in the affluent West.

Cancer remains one of the major unresolved human issues of our time. A dispassionate account of this highly emotive subject is here presented with a view to enabling interested readers to make up their minds what to do about their own mode of life. The choice lies between either doing nothing, that is, continuing to delude oneself in the midst of painfully tangible evidence to the contrary that cancer is something that can affect others, but which just could not *possibly* happen to oneself, or alternatively trying to minimise the cancer risks by resolving to re-think and to re-model one's own way of life along the more austere lines advocated in this book. The personal motivation that this will require should be generated by the mere thought that what is at stake is nothing less than one's own personal survival, surely a sufficiently potent incentive for putting up with the occasionally irksome restrictions of a more disciplined life-style.

When a man is drowning and there is a lifebelt at hand, you throw it to him — you do not waste time considering whether it is the right size and shape whilst he goes under, perhaps for the third time. To the question, asked by many, whether there is sufficient proof concerning primary cancer prevention, the answer must be that we have adequate evidence on which to act *now*. There is still much testing to be done but we possess sufficient knowledge to say that those who disregard what we already know about the consequences of an imprudent diet, excessive alcoholic consumption, heavy cigarette smoking and easy sex do so at their peril.

2 DIET

It is tragically ironic that the appalling cancer death toll is largely unnecessary, because in the present state of medical knowledge cancer can be shown to be preventable in about half of the patients currently dying from it. Paradoxically, therein lies the brightest hope for avoiding such carnage in the future.

In practice, the effective application of this recent knowledge to the community depends for success on the wholehearted participation of society as a whole, but this participation is not forthcoming because there are very few in today's consumer society who, while still fit, healthy or young, would willingly forego the culinary and sensual delights that result from over-indulgence in food and drinks, etc. This over-indulgence has become one of today's most popular rituals to which everyone readily subscribes, including doctors, elected representatives of successive governments and others in public life, who really should be giving an exemplary lead.

This is the more regrettable because of the mounting evidence which shows that, although cancer is of multi-factorial origin and although the precipitant factors encompass such wide-ranging phenomena as the effects of hormones, chronic irritation, ageing, immunological status, stress and psychological state, over half of the more common forms of cancer are related to *diet*, which makes the combined effect of food and drink a more important determinant of the risk of cancer than even smoking.

In Western society we seem to be doing something right with regard to preventing the development of stomach cancer and something very wrong in regard to putting ourselves at a very high risk in relation to two other forms of cancer, namely cancer of the breast and cancer of the bowel.

These two forms of cancer always seem to go together in the affluent Western countries, where they are common, and where they are associated with low rates of cancer of the stomach. These low rates appear to be related to a reduced intake of salt-pickled, smoked and spiced foods as well as total absence in Western diet of such culinary Japanese 'delicacies' as stomach-cancer-inducing bracken fern, hot rice-gruel, soya-bean sauce, Sake, asbestos-related talc-like food additives and the deliberate charring of fish and rice until the outer side is black.

11

Conversely the *high* rates of cancer of the stomach in Japan are associated with *low* rates of the other two forms of cancer probably because the Western type of diet, when compared with that of Japan, contains more red meat, animal fat (butter, cream, bacon), cholesterol (egg-yolk) and refined carbohydrates (white bakery products, sugar) and less dietary fibre.

It is thus not surprising that Japanese who migrate from their native land to Hawaii or California and who become westernised in their dietary habits can expect to assume within only one or two generations the disease-characteristics of their new country of adoption. In other words their incidence of stomach cancer will decrease, whereas the mortality rates of the other two forms of cancer will approach those of their host country.

The enormous increase in the twentieth century of degenerative diseases in the sophisticated communities is unquestionably due to Western eating habits. Not only do we eat double the calories needed but compared with the under-privileged nations we consume seven times as much fat, six times as much sugar and about ten times as much cholesterol, whilst we eat very little in the way of starchy or fibre-rich foods. During both World War I and World War II degenerative diseases in food-rationed countries decreased, as they also did in prisoner-of-war camps and concentration camps. This beneficial dietary effects, which were most pronounced in meat and dairy-producing countries (where land-use was changed to grain production) can be attributed to the complete absence of fat in the meagre war-rations.

What seems to determine the different eating patterns in the various countries of the world is not only availability of food and the local traditional customs and habits but also religious commands and spiritual beliefs. For instance, in contrast to the diet ordinarily eaten by the British, Central Europeans and the Americans, Seventh Day Adventists, who are an evangelical religious group with about 2.5 million members worldwide and 500,000 in North America, follow a lacto-ovo-vegetarian diet: in addition most of them avoid alcohol, coffee, tea, hot condiments and spices. This austere regime has proved to be of great benefit to health in that the relatively low fat and cholesterol content of the diet in association with its high cellulose-fibre content has had a favourable influence on the physiology of the gut. This has resulted in low cancer rates, due to a rapid transit time of stools through the gut, a low output of bile acids (substances which are potentially convertible to carcinogens) and an altered type of intestinal bacteria with reduced metabolic activity.

Again conversely, our ordinary Western type of diet with its characteristic small hard stools is associated firstly with a prolonged transit time of stools; secondly with a very high bile acid content; and thirdly with a change in bacterial flora which is characterised by bacteria with a specially active metabolic capacity.

These three factors may be responsible for the recent startling increase in bowel cancer which can be explained in terms of hyperactive bacteria, interacting with the cancer-producing (carcinogenic) break-down products of the plentiful bile acids, to produce a carcinogenic substance which as a result of its prolonged contact with the bowel wall will continue to irritate the wall-lining and will eventually induce malignant change.

It is this same high-fat, low-fibre type of Western diet, in particular dairy products high in (the enzyme Lactase requiring) milk-fat, such as butter, cheese, cream and whole-milk, which also indirectly exerts an adverse effect on the breast, by creating conditions in the bowel that are favourable to the production of oestrogenic hormones and by stimulating the pituitary gland to secrete Prolactin. Increased levels of these hormones circulating in the blood will continue to irritate existing pre-malignant lesions in the breast which under this influence may undergo malignant change.

It is most important to increase stool bulk and softness by consuming a great deal of roughage in the form of unabsorbable high-residue cellulose fibre. This is achieved by eating a great deal of fruit, vegetables, cereals, full-grain bread and, in particular, unprocessed bran of which at least two heaped tablespoonfuls daily are mandatory.

Since deficiencies of Vitamin A and Vitamin C have been shown to enhance the susceptibility to various forms of cancer the amount of Vitamin A consumed should be boosted by eating lots of green and yellow vegetables, in particular Brussels sprouts, cabbage and cauliflower, as well as carrots. Vegetables should be consumed together with large amounts of Vitamin C-containing fresh fruit, in particular oranges.

Since both Vitamin A and Vitamin C levels in the body must not be allowed to fall, Vitamin C should be taken regularly in the form of ascorbic acid tablets and Vitamin A in the form of halibut oil capsules, when insufficient fruit and vegetables are eaten.

Dietary Fibre

Neither sugar nor fat contains any dietary fibre whatever. In other words they have none of the high-residue roughage contained in wholemeal bread, bran, breakfast cereals, pulses, fruit and vegetables. This means that at least 60 per cent of the food-energy eaten every day is totally devoid of roughage even though dietary fibre is the *only* component of food with a low calorie content and therefore not fattening.

Obese people, as well as looking less attractive, have a higher risk of developing degenerative illnesses such as diabetes or heart disease, so there is every good reason to strive to stay slim. This can best be achieved with the help of fibre-rich food because a substantial part of it remains unavailable for digestion and so decreases (by 2 per cent) the amount of food-energy that is actually absorbed. The indigestible portion is expedited as unabsorbable roughage straight through the bowel. As a result of its heavy bulk it easily provides the 200g of roughage necessary to trigger off the emptying reflex in the rectum, and because of its soft consistency it is much more rapidly excreted, thereby combating constipation and with it, a host of other illnesses. Additionally, its bulky volume increases and prolongs the 'full-up' feeling and reduces the desire for food. For instance high-residue, fibre-rich wholemeal bread is much more filling than soft, fibre-depleted white bread, white cake or white biscuits. This is also the reason why fibre-rich, starchy potatoes (either boiled or baked in their jackets) contrary to general opinion, are *not* fattening, provided they are eaten without butter or margarine, and not cooked in oil.

Fats and sugars are needed solely as a source of energy for heavy physical work and for athletic pursuits. In the absence of such physical activities regular excessive intake of fat and/or sugar will inevitably lead to fat storage and weight gain. This is why 40 per cent of the Western population are over-weight and 30 per cent try, unsuccessfully, to slim at least once a year. In the process they spend annually £40 million in the UK and £350 million in the USA on slimming cures.

Even for superbly fit people there is no dietetic 'carte blanche' which would allow them to eat and drink with impunity because they soon lose the low blood viscosity and high blood-flow velocity characteristic of athletes, which affords such remarkable protection against degenerative diseases.

Few people realise that 10 per cent of most sweetened soft drinks is composed of sugar; that alcoholic drinks are fattening; in fact that 20 per cent of the calories eaten in a day come from sugar and almost 40 per cent from fat.

It is also worth remembering that a piece of cake (composed of fat and sugar) contains twice the number of calories lost in a jog of 45 minutes.

Most people have been brought up from infancy almost exclusively on low-fibre, high energy foods containing much fat and sugar which lead to many degenerative diseases. Fortunately today there is widespread awareness that a high-fibre diet is both healthy and slimming.

Despite this, when it comes to changing lifelong eating habits, few can bring themselves to forego the old accustomed over-indulgence in the wrong kind of food and drink.

So it must be emphasised again: bran, unrefined cereals, wholemeal bread, whole wheat flour, unpolished rice, vegetables, fruit, fish, poultry, skimmed milk and low fat cheeses should be eaten regularly because they do not clog up the arteries. What should be *severely restricted or avoided altogether* is butter, cream, fatty meats, fried food, unskimmed milk, high fat cheeses, mayonnaise, ice cream, sugar, confectionery, cake and alcohol. All these foods have a high fat and/or sugar content. This increases blood viscosity and slows down blood velocity and so pre-disposes to tissue breakdown, premature ageing and a poor quality of life.

Eating vegetables, fruit and high-fibre foods will not only supply far fewer calories but by virtue of their bulk will tend to prolong the 'full-up' feeling thus reducing appetite and promoting intestinal peristalsis. This is very important because constipation is still one of the commonest disabilities in the affluent West and aperients remain in such great demand that each year £4 million are spent on laxatives in Great Britain and £35 million in the USA.

The total daily intake of fats should be reduced to about 80 grams which means that much less than 3 ounces (84 grams) of butter should be eaten every day. Instead of butter, a low fat margarine should be used and polyunsaturated vegetable oils such as sunflower or corn oil are preferable for cooking.

Skimmed milk should replace whole milk because cream is particularly unhealthy. Cottage cheese or skimmed milk cheeses should be eaten in preference to whole milk cheeses and sorbets should replace whole milk ice cream; rich or creamy chocolate desserts should be avoided, as should strong coffee.

Meat should be trimmed of all visible fat. Grilling and steaming is better than frying and roasting, which means that one should reduce the frequency of eating fried fish and chips.

The intake of cholesterol should be limited to 300 mg daily. Since one egg-yolk contains 235 mg of cholesterol, not more than four visible eggs per week should be eaten. Mainly the egg-white, which contains all the goodness, should be used and the egg-yolk should be rejected. For cooking, egg-substitute should be employed.

Meats that are lowest in cholesterol content are veal, chicken and turkey. These are preferable to red meats but even then fish is by far the most wholesome food and should replace meat and poultry as often as possible.

The amount of processed, prepacked convenience foods, which are high in empty calories (low in nutrition,) should be reduced to a minimum, as should chocolates and refined sugar.

Because of the health-promoting effect of food rich in dietary fibre it is particularly regrettable that the daily wholemeal bread and potato consumption has been severely reduced. In 1870 it averaged 400g of wholemeal bread and 300g of potatoes (providing a daily total of 40g of fibre, 8g in the form of crude fibre). By 1970 it has dropped to only 200g of *white* bread and 200g of potatoes (yielding a total of 10g of fibre, no more than 2g in the form of crude fibre). This is exactly one quarter of the dietary roughage eaten one hundred years ago.

The ill-effects of such fibre-depleted diet are compounded by the concurrent reversal of the relative proportions of fats and sugar on the one hand and of starches on the other that are eaten today. Whereas in 1870 only 20 per cent of our food-energy came from sugar and fats (the remaining 80 per cent being provided by cereals and potatoes) now 60 per cent or more of our food-energy comes from eating fats and sugar and less than 40 per cent from cereals and potatoes. The increasing incidence in the twentieth century of diet-related degenerative diseases in our overfed third of the world is a direct consequence of such uniformed and undiscriminating food selection.

This adverse trend is readily reversible by a simple change in dietary habits exemplified for instance by a switch from whole milk to skimmed milk (or always giving the top of the milk to the cat!) or, by habitually having fruit or low-fat yoghurt for a dessert instead of pudding, cake or fruit-pie.

3 NUTRIENTS

There are two main reasons for eating; of these the first is concerned with the provision of nutrients, for tissue growth and repair, for muscular activity and for chemical reactions in the body. The second reason, rarely conducive to good health, but for many a more pleasurable one is that we eat for *fun*. Since we eat food, not nutrients, we need to know which of the three main types of food i.e. proteins, fats and carbohydrates are most required for good health.

Proteins

These are to be found mainly in meat, fish, dairy products and cereals. In fact, proteins are the only *really* essential nutrients because they are needed for tissue growth and repair and since the body is unable to synthesise them, about 10 per cent of our food intake should be in the form of proteins.

Fats

The most commonly eaten fats are butter, margarine, cooking fats, salad oils, mayonnaise and dairy cream. *All* fats are not only unnecessary but can actually be harmful, particularly when eaten to excess.

Carbohydrates

These are comprised of: 1) sugars, which are simple carbohydrates; 2) starchy foods, which are more complex. Starchy carbohydrates such as wholemeal bread or potatoes provide some of the important dietary fibre required for the proper functioning of the intestines and are thus essential for good health, but *sugar* is totally without nutritional value *in whatever form it is taken* — white sugar, brown sugar, raw sugar, Demerera sugar, molasses, syrup, honey, jam, marmalade, orangeade, lemonade, Cola, cakes, puddings, biscuits, chocolate, sweets or ice-cream — what we are actually eating is *sugar*, chemically pure but full of fattening calories. This refined sugar, it must be stressed, is completely unnecessary for good health because the little the body needs is amply supplied in a simpler and healthier form in fruit and milk.

Vitamins

Much evidence has accumulated of late on the protective action against cancer afforded by high levels of Vitamin A in the body. More than three-quarters of Vitamin A in the British diet come preformed as retinol from the liver, from some dairy products, and from vitamin pills. The remainder comes directly from carrots, or from green leafy or yellow vegetables which yield carotin or other carotenoids which can be split into Vitamin A in the intestine.

Similarly Vitamin C has been found to have a protective action against cancer. Hence the great importance of eating plentiful fresh fruit, salads and vegetables. When fruit and vegetables are not available and therefore eaten in less than adequate amounts the vitamin levels in the body should be supplemented by consumption of vitamin tablets obtainable at pharmacies as ascorbic acid (Vitamin C) and halibut oil capsules (Vitamin A).

This new pharmacological approach to the prevention of cancer is called *chemo-prevention* and relies on pharmacological enhancement of intrinsic physiological mechanisms intended to arrest or prevent development of malignant cells. In order to be effective, chemo-prevention must be applied during the pre-malignant stages of the disease: that is, before cancer actually begins.

No-one eating a mixed diet of proteins, starchy carbohydrates, vegetables and fruit should need any vitamin or mineral supplements in tablet form.

In any case one carrot contains a three days' supply of Vitamin A which is also plentiful in yellow fruit and green vegetables. Well-fed people have about a two years' supply of Vitamin A in their livers.

The Vitamin B complex, consisting of half a dozen different vitamins, is found in cereals, yeast and in pulses (peas, beans, lentils).

Half an orange contains one day's supply of Vitamin C which is also found in fresh fruit and vegetables.

Milk and cheeses are rich in Vitamin D, as are cod-liver and herrings.

A small breakfast-portion of bran, whole wheat or wheat germ contains an adequately protective amount of Vitamin E. Wheat germ, sunflower seeds and avocados are rich in Vitamin F, as is evening primrose oil.

Minerals

All of the most important minerals are plentiful in a mixed diet and so there is never any likelihood of a shortage. They include: calcium (found in milk and cheeses), phosphorus (contained in poultry and sausages), magnesium (present in bran and nuts), iron (contained in curry powder, red meat, liver and baked beans) and zinc (present in meat, offal and shellfish) and selenium (found in seafood, yeast, garlic, onions and mushrooms).

Fruit and Vegetables

Apart from containing Vitamin C, fruit and most vegetables have no other appreciable nutritional value, but being rich in dietary fibre they are filling and so tend to reduce appetite and the risk of obesity. Even more important, they are bulky, and by promoting active bowel peristalsis help to reduce constipation.

Rice

Rice (naturally brown rice) should be cooked in a pressure cooker in as little water as possible in order not to leach out the Vitamin B. The water should not be discarded but used for cooking.

Potatoes

Potatoes, a starchy food with 2 per cent protein and 80 per cent water, contain Vitamins B and C. It should be noted that the Vitamin C is destroyed when:

    a) potatoes are cooked in a copper vessel;
    b) they are kept hot for a long period;
    c) they are re-heated;

d) the water in which they are to be cooked has not been boiled first to remove the oxygen;
e) they are cooked in too little water, which encourages the presence of oxygen;
f) they are cooked with baking soda.

It should be emphasised that potatoes are not fattening provided that they are boiled, or baked and eaten in their jackets without butter, oil or margarine.

Bread

A standard 500g loaf contains 250g starch, 50g protein and 10g fat; the rest is water. It is often called a starchy food, which of course it is, but it also provides an adequate amount of protein — in fact from the point of view of *protein* we could live on bread alone. Bread made of wholemeal flour contains 100 per cent wheat grain of which 8.5 per cent is fibre, whereas bread made of white flour has lost 30 per cent during milling and thus has only 70 per cent of the wheat grain and no fibre-rich bran at all. Yet white bread continues to capture 60 per cent of the market sales and wholemeal bread only 30 per cent! Brown bread with 0.6 per cent of fibre captures 10 per cent of the market.

In summary, a well-balanced mixed diet provides added protection against cancer when it contains, as it invariably does, adequate amounts of Vitamins A, C, E, and of selenium, because all four, on account of their oxidation-blocking action, are protective against oxidative cell-damage, which is thought to initiate the malignant change in the cell's DNA (a protein made by the cell with the help of enzymes, which determines the cell's behaviour).

4 CALORIES

In practice the only effective method of controlling weight is by counting calories. Calories are measuring units which indicate the amount of energy contained in an item of food. A few practical examples might aid better understanding: we consume 100 calories by eating either 1 slice of bread and butter, or a ¼lb (113g) of spaghetti, or a ¼lb (113g) of haddock; 1 whole water melon, or 1 banana; 2 cauliflowers, 2 cucumbers, 8 lettuces or 10 tomatoes. Similarly we absorb 100 calories when we drink a half-pint of beer, a glass of wine, a small sherry or a single whisky. In addition alcohol may stimulate appetite. Whereas a boiled potato contains only 75 calories, ten chips contain 140 calories. Sweets contain by weight six times the calories of boiled potatoes and eight times the calories of raw apples, yet they are completely devoid of nutritional value.

The calories content of food can be readily calculated: each gram of fat yields 9 calories, each gram of alcohol 7 calories, each gram of protein and each gram of sugar 4 calories respectively. From this it is very obvious that fat has the highest calorie content per volume and that eating butter and margarine, or constantly frying foods in cooking fats or oil will immeasurably increase calorie absorption; a percentage of these surplus calories not needed to fuel the body with energy is then stored as body fat and this is what makes people overweight.

Calories are not only used to calculate energy *absorbed*; they also serve as units to measure energy *expended*. The simple effort of merely staying alive requires a non-stop energy supply for all the biological processes taking place in the body. For instance, in any one day, calories are required for over 100,000 heartbeats and for more than 60,000 breaths.

Calories are expended to keep the brain functioning and to maintain the continuous snake-like peristaltic movement of the bowel. They are needed to keep up the body temperature and used on the exchange of fluids as they pass in and out of the body cells. Even in bed, calories are consumed at the rate of one per minute: nearly 500 are used up in a night of 8 hours sleep.

Muscular activity, however, requires by far the most calories. We use 2 calories per minute when sitting and writing; 3 when driving a car; 5 when walking quickly or polishing a floor; 7 playing tennis, 10 digging or shovelling, 11 cycling fast, 14 swimming vigorously and 20 when running upstairs.

The average daily calorie requirement for an active adult male is thought to be in the region of 3,000. The greatest consumption, as would be expected, is during the 8-hour working day, when half of the total is used. The 8-hour leisure period needs another 1,000 calories and finally, about 500 are used up during the night. It is interesting to note that for an active adult female, the figures are lower. She requires only 2,300 calories and consumes 1,000 at work, 900 at leisure and 400 at night.

Weight Gain

It is not unusual for some women to gain about 44lb (20kg) in the 20 years between the age of 35, when the average weight is 132lb (60kg), and 55 when it is 176lb (80kg). How imperceptibly this increase comes about will be more readily understood when it is realised that *one* extra slice of bread and butter a day can contribute an extra 100 calories a day. This represents an extra weight gain of 3 grams a day and repeated daily this will work out at more than 20 gram a week or 2lb (1kg) a year. All this from only one extra slice of bread and butter a day!

If you continue to eat the same amount of food year after year you will gradually gain weight as you grow older because with age the body requires less energy to satisfy its metabolic needs. Additionally, physical activity usually decreases after young adulthood, and if the food intake remains constant, the resultant weight gain will also be constant. Because of the serious risk of obesity to health, life insurance companies charge overweight people much higher premiums; from their records it appears that the life expectancy of a person who at the age of 45 is 26lb (12kg) overweight is reduced by 25 per cent and that he or she is likely to die at the age of 60 instead of 80.

It should be emphasised that it is infinitely simpler to maintain weight than to try to lose it once gained. As an example: to lose 1kg a week, the total daily food energy intake must be reduced by at least 1,000 calories and this requires tremendous motivation and a will-power of iron. To be more specific, to lose 1 g of fat the food intake must be reduced by 7 calories; therefore, if the desired weekly weight loss is to be 1kg (and it is unwise, and invariably unsuccessful in the long run, to attempt a more rapid loss of weight) the usual food intake must be cut by 1,000 calories a day. Such drastic reduction in energy consumed results in a daily loss of 150g. If maintained every day this will result in a loss of 1kg in a full week.

So to lose weight it is important to count the calories in *every* item of food. A tablespoon of mayonnaise, for instance, has more than twice the calories of a tablespoon of pure sugar and a tablespoon of ketchup has about the same number of calories as a teaspoon of sugar. A ham sandwich has 300 calories, a meringue pie 420, and a steak pudding 600.

5 DIETARY MYTHS

There probably exist more preconceived ideas, superstitions and prejudices on the subject of food than on any other topic of corresponding popularity. Some of these misconceptions have been handed down from generation to generation, others have been misleadingly publicised by the media and even more have arisen as a result of unscrupulously slanted and profit-motivated commercial advertising. The following paragraphs attempt to explode some of the myths, to correct some of the misapprehensions and to fill in some of the deliberate omissions.

Biscuits

It is never stated in advertisements promoting special brands of biscuits that they contain the uniquely unhealthy combination of pure fat and refined sugar! Nor is it stressed that because of this they are totally lacking in nutriment and that if eaten regularly their high content of empty calories must inevitably lead to a gain in weight.

Cakes

Similarly, it is an intentionally misleading psychological manipulation for commercial ends that links home-making with baking a cake. What is not mentioned is that during cake-baking the nutritious flour which contains 10 per cent of protein is degraded, first by sugar which contains no protein, and then further diluted by fat, which also contains no protein. This means that the resulting flour-confectionery is much less nutritious than the original flour and may even be harmful by contributing to obesity.

Honey

There is an aura of romance and magic surrounding the beneficial effects of honey. Contrary to most honey-lovers' deeply held conviction, honey is nothing more than refined sugar (fructose), which may well please the palate but which, although more slowly absorbed than ordinary sugar, serves no other useful medical purpose.

Similarly the assumed magical effect of bees' Royal Jelly, alleged to have a rejuvenating effect, is totally false. Admittedly the Royal Jelly transforms worker bees into queen bees but, considering the size of a bee, the relative dose for a human being would have to be 20 tons and that presupposes that one would wish to be transformed into a queen bee!

Yoghurt

This is another food with alleged 'magical' properties! It should be explained that the intestine is the natural home of micro-organisms which help in the formation of stools; these putrefactive bacteria, according to ancient myth, were alleged to have a shortening effect on one's lifespan.

Because yoghurt contains different, that is souring, bacteria, it was thought that these would neutralise the stool's own 'life-shortening' bacteria and in this way prolong life. A good story, but totally untrue, as myths usually are!

Sea-salt

A great deal has been claimed about the superiority of sea-salt over ordinary cooking salt; it also contains a small amount of Vitamin B_{12} and of iodine, but in a non-landlocked country there is an ample supply of iodine in the normal food anyway. Otherwise sea-salt only contains impurities of sea-water and is therefore medically valueless and, at the same time, much more expensive.

Vitamin E

This Vitamin is available in adequate amounts in most natural foods and therefore no supplement is necessary.

Being an anti-oxidant, it is thought in some quarters to be useful as an anti-carcinogenic protective factor by neutralising cancer-inducing oxygen radicals in the body. Contrary to popular belief it does not promote fertility.

Organically Grown Food

Organic manure and fertilisers in the form of animal droppings, compost, blood meal, hoof and horn meal, as used by old-fashioned gardeners, can be utilised by nature only after these substances have been broken down into their basic chemical constituents, namely potash, phosphate and sulphate of ammonia. These three substances are in fact the main ingredients of the so-called inorganic or chemical fertilisers. The only conceivable advantage of natural, organic manure and compost is that they loosen up the soil and release their chemical constituents gradually.

Meat

It is not correct, as claimed by many butchers, that the most tender portions of meat are the fat cuts. Whereas lean meat contains only 5 per cent fat with 20 per cent protein and 75 per cent water, meat as sold on the slab has 50 per cent of fat. Neither is it true that the white meat of poultry is more nutritious than red meat. What *is* true is that poultry, being leaner, contains less fat and cholesterol, and is therefore healthier. Although fat meat is not quickly digested because the fat delays emptying of the stomach and thus increases the 'full-up' feeling, a healthy stomach has no difficulty in digesting fat. Nevertheless all fat should be cut off the meat before cooking and should never be eaten.

Hung Meat

What makes meat tough is its indigestible fibrous tissue. Hunted animals produce quantities of lactic acid just prior to death, due to intense muscular activity. This acid gelatinises the fibres and tenderises the meat. Farm animals, slaughtered whilst standing still, give less tender meat, but acids continue to form after death in the muscles and that is why hung meat becomes more tender with time.

Free-range Meat

There is some controversy about the food-value of free-range meat compared with stall-fed meat. Both are equally nutritious but feed-lots produce fat meat whereas free-range meat is much leaner; in fact farmers already have the knowledge (but are reluctant to use it because it would be commercially less profitable), to raise cow-breeds with low-fat milk and low-fat meat. The priceless benefits for the public that would accrue from these specially bred fatless cattle-species would include sausages, hamburgers and hot dogs with lean meat, and dairy products with low saturated-fat content.

Barbecues

Charcoal-grilling of steaks at barbecues, until the outside of the meat is charred black, can produce powerful carcinogens in the areas subjected to the very high temperatures and should be avoided because these carcinogens are known to produce cancer in animals. However, good cooks do not usually burn much of the food they are cooking, although they may caramelise it. In normal circumstances the temperatures involved in barbecue cooking rarely exceed 200° C, which is quite safe.

Meat and Health

Better health is not, as frequently stated, the result of greater meat consumption. It is due to a balanced diet consisting of proteins, minerals and vitamins.

Eating more meat puts an extra burden on the kidneys. Even though healthy kidneys are perfectly able to excrete the resulting greatly increased amounts of nitrogen, there are three potentially harmful side effects that such a high meat consumption entails.

1) The toxic by-products of increased protein metabolism, such as uric acid, urea and ammonia, when present in excess, can contribute to arthritis and other illnesses.

2) If all the protein eaten by the high meat consumption is not used up for energy, the excess will be stored as fat.

3) Since all animal protein is rich in cholesterol, increased meat consumption will be harmful to people with a predisposition to heart disease and high blood pressure. Since we cannot tell in advance who is and who is not so predisposed, it is best to restrict the intake of meat at all times.

Slimming Cures

It is understandable that in the search for the quickest slimming 'cures' even more intelligent people become gullible and put their faith in all kinds of magical diets. Some, for example, believe that as long as they start each meal with a grapefruit, they can eat as much as they wish during the subsequent meal without gaining weight! Of course, this is nonsense.

Another misconception is that a limit of two meals a day will ensure a loss of weight. The truth is that it is the *calorie content* of the food which is the determining factor. Provided that the total eaten is the same, *five small meals* are more slimming than two large ones, because at each meal some of the consumed energy is dissipated in the form of heat.

Slimming is helped by eating slowly and masticating well. This causes more saliva to be formed which helps to fill the stomach; by eating slowly one might therefore well eat less.

There are three main reasons why cigarettes help to keep smokers slim. Firstly smoking depresses appetite and a smoker therefore tends to eat less; then it speeds up digestion so there is less time for fat to be absorbed and stored. Finally, each cigarette releases sugar into the bloodstream, so there is no desire for sugar and other sweet foods.

Conversely, once smoking is given up, all these weight-reducing factors are reversed: the appetite increases, digestion is slowed down, and occasionally there is an irresistible craving for sugar. The result is a rapid weight gain in the initial period after giving up the habit and it sometimes takes the body at least six months to re-adjust to the absence of the noxious, though weight-reducing, effects of cigarettes.

A direct causal relationship seems to exist between the frequency of bowel cancer and the consumption of meat. In Tibet and Thailand very little meat is eaten and bowel cancer is virtually unknown. Meat consumption is modest in Japan and Chile, and so is bowel cancer incidence. The largest amount of meat is eaten in Canada, Scotland, Australia and New Zealand, countries with the greatest number of bowel cancer victims.

6 ALCOHOL

Alcoholism is a historical disease which can be traced back thousands of years. It has shown a constant pattern of 'ups and downs' and currently we are in the midst of one of the greatest, if not the greatest 'up', ever known in history. In America, Britain and Europe, particularly in France and Russia, it is a very serious problem indeed. The sinister part of the upward surge is the fact that the increased figures in recent years come largely from women and, even more sadly, children.

Alcoholism is of course part of the universal drug problem, because alcohol is a drug. The heavy drugs get great publicity in all the media, although they are really far less important than alcohol because for every one sufferer from addictive drugs there are twenty alcoholics in the world.

Alcholism is an insidious illness which progresses in a most sinister way. It is not only a physical condition; there are aspects of it which are mental, social and moral, and its repercussions extend beyond the alcoholic to the wife or husband, family, friends and fellow workers. Furthermore, alcoholism is responsible not only for much of the violence, hooliganism and vandalism seen today, but also for accidents, many of them fatal, which occur on the road, at work and in the home.

Persons employed in the drinking trade, such as French vineyard workres, publicans, commercial travellers in spirits and brewery workers have a much greater incidence of cancer affecting the upper air and digestive passages. For instance the highest incidence of cancer of the oesophagus in Europe is found in Britanny and Normandy where ciders and cider-based liqueurs are produced locally. Besides increasing proneness to cancer, regular over-consumption of alcohol also causes liver cirrhosis, brain degeneration and pre-senile dementia as well as premature loss of sex drive.

It is a sad reflection on public enlightenment that the majority of alcoholics are not just vagrants; many are in the executive ranks of business and in the professions, and include quite a considerable number of doctors.

It is frequently forgotten that alcohol is a high-energy food which passes straight through the blood into the fat stores. There are over 70 calories in a half-pint of beer or a small glass of sherry, 90 calories in a glass of wine and 130 calories in a single whisky.

It is not unusual for the average person when invited out, or sometimes even when dining at home, to have two single or one double whisky before a meal, three glasses of wine during a meal and a small brandy after a meal. This relatively moderate amount of alcohol adds a total of 650 calories to the food consumed, which is equivalent to having eaten a second meal.

This additional energy, if it has to be used up, would necessitate 2 hours of brisk walking, 1 hour of fast cycling or 45 minutes of energetic swimming, for without this physical exertion these 650 calories would inevitably be converted into a weight gain.

There are five mimportant guidelines which should govern the amount of alcohol that can be safely consumed.

1) The type of drink is irrelevant.
2) What matters is the alcohol content of the drink.
3) Half a pint of beer is equivalent in alcoholic content to one glass of sherry or wine, or to one small whisky or gin.
4) Three pints of beer (or its equivalent, that is six glasses of wine or sherry, or six small whiskies or gins) if drunk at once is too much because it not only raises the alcoholic content of the blood above the legally permissible level for driving but also because if taken regularly it will eventually lead to alcoholic dependence.
5) Four pints of beer (or its equivalent in alcoholic content, that is eight glasses of wine or sherry, or eight small whiskies or gins) when taken regularly inevitably damage one's health and must eventually lead to addiction, that is chronic alcoholism; an 'occasional binge' does little harm.

Immoderate consumption of alcohol is particularly damaging if it is associated with cigarette smoking. The two seem to interact, i.e. each potentiates the effect of the other and can often cause cancers of the mouth, pharynx, larynx and oesophagus.

Alcohol-induced illnesses, particularly fatty degeneration of the liver leading to fatal liver cirrhosis, as already stated, affect all social classes including the executive ranks of business and the professions, especially the medical profession.

7 CIGARETTE SMOKING

Every year 100,000 victims (that is one person every 5 minutes) die unnecessarily from the results of heavy smoking. There is ample and totally irrefutable evidence of the disastrous effects of cigarette smoking on health. The three noxious components of tobacco responsible for the damage are: tar, nicotine and carbon monoxide.

1) The tar in the cigarette causes lung cancer; it also causes the deadly emphysema, chronic bronchitis and bladder cancer.

2) The nicotine, by producing an anaesthetic-like state of mental tranquillity and relaxation, yet at the same time by releasing adrenalin and sugar which makes the smoker feel alert and ready to cope with any emergency, becomes addictive and is responsible for the continuous craving experienced by smokers.

3) The carbon monoxide concentration (higher in cigarettes with filters) causes hardening of the arteries by putting up the blood level of the low density constituent of the blood fat called cholesterol. This gets deposited in the walls of damaged blood vessels which ultimately become blocked by these deposits, thus cutting off the blood supply and causing death of a part of vital organs, such as the heart (coronary thrombosis) or the brain (stroke).

Since contraceptive pills increase the clotting tendency of the blood, women over the age of 35 taking the pill who are also regular smokers run a much higher risk of cerebral thrombosis and should cease smoking.

There follow two examples of the great benefit to general health of giving up smoking.

1) It can be shown that in the absence of smoking the incidence of lung cancer will drop by 95 per cent and the incidence of all other forms of cancer will be reduced by 40 per cent within only one generation.

2) In 1951 Professor Sir Richard Doll of Oxford recorded the smoking habits of 35,000 British doctors. By 1966 the lung cancer death rates among the general population aged 35 to 64 had risen by 7 per cent whereas among British doctors, many of whom had given up smoking, the lung cancer death rate over the same period had fallen by 38 per cent.

The findings not only confirmed that smoking caused lung cancer, they also indicated that general discontinuance of the smoking habit would lower the number of deaths from the disease: in other words, it always pays, however late in the day, to give up or to reduce smoking.

With women smokers, statistics showed that in 1960 the death rate from lung cancer was 5 per hundred thousand. By 1975 due to heavier smoking the figure had trebled to 15 per hundred thousand. Similarly, comparing cancer death rates in the two sexes: in 1960, for each woman dying of lung cancer there were seven men; by 1975, due to the heavier smoking by women, the ratio was reduced to three male deaths to each female death.

Non-smoking wives of heavy smokers have a higher risk of developing lung cancer and this risk is the higher the greater the number of cigarettes smoked. What is more, in countries where only a small proportion of women smoke, the effect of passive 'smoking' on lung cancer in women actually becomes more important than that of direct smoking.

A 14-year study of 265,000 Japanese men and women concluded that a husband who smoked 20 cigarettes a day doubled a non-smoking wife's risk of dying of lung cancer.

Heavy smoking is also known to increase significantly the incidence of chronic bronchitis, strokes, conorary thrombosis, hypertension, arteriosclerosis, cancer of the stomach, cancer of the bladder and, in conjunction with alcohol, cancer of the oesophagus and cancer of the other upper air and digestive passages.

Do not smoke at all. If however, you cannot give up cigarettes, it is relatively harmless to smoke up to six a day, always provided that only half of each cigarette is smoked and, in particular provided that the smoke is not inhaled.

For those wishing to give up smoking there is a nicotine-containing chewing gum, which makes weaning somewhat less difficult by decreasing the persistent craving for nicotine. Each time the smoker wants to give in and reaches for another cigarette, he will be able to take (and suck) a small piece of chewing gum instead. Since the nicotine in the chewing gum will enter the blood directly from the mouth, the lungs will be totally bypassed and thus spared, yet the continued presence of nicotine in the tissues will mute the otherwise irresistible craving for yet another cigarette.

8 OTHER TYPES OF CANCER AND THEIR PREVENTION

Cancer of the Penis

Cancer of the penis can be prevented by total circumcision at birth and in those not circumcised by regular, thorough washing behind the foreskin, with warm water and soap. For this to be possible the foreskin must be retractable; if it is not, an operation is mandatory since a non-retractable foreskin predisposes to cancer as a result of the chronic irritation and inflammation set up by the secretion trapped behind the foreskin.

In this context it is highly relevant that cancer of the penis is not seen in Parsees, an enlightened sect of Persians, now living in India, who do not practise circumcision but with their religion based on purity they are particularly meticulous in their personal hygiene and thus remain free of the disease.

Cancer of the Cervix

Cancer of the neck of the womb (cervix) seems to be related to the sexual act, since the disease spares nuns and virgins. It is common in prostitutes and the risk of developing it increases with the number of marriages. It is extremely rare in Parsees and in Jewesses.

It is inversely related to the age at which sexual intercourse first takes place. In other words, the younger the teenager, the greater the risk of contracting the disease. This risk is further increased by sexual promiscuity, again especially in the 'teens when the cervix is very vulnerable to injury, and by having a venereal infection, particularly if contracted early in life.

There is increasing evidence that the use of barrier contraceptives is of great protective value because the disease is apparently of venereal origin due to sexually transmitted infection with the Herpes Virus Type II, or the Genital Wart Virus, which is usually passed from the infected uncircumcised male during intercourse.

The risk of contracting cancer of the neck of the womb can be greatly reduced by:

1) postponing the beginning of regular intercourse until well beyond the 'teens;

2) using a barrier contraceptive;

3) having a single partner;

4) making one's partner, especially if uncircumcised, wash thoroughly behind the foreskin before intercourse;

5) having a hot bath immediately after coitus, with particularly meticulous cleansing of the vagina. This is an additional simple measure of immense protective value.

Though not related to the sexual act the risk of contracting cancer of the uterine body is greater in obese women. Many fat people eat no more than many thin people, so obesity cannot be ascribed entirely to sloth and gluttony. Nevertheless the laws of thermodynamics apply to women as much as to steam engines and the body cannot store energy as fat unless its intake of energy exceeds its output.

Cancer of the breast

The breast appears particularly prone to react to excessive milk-fat consumption, in that breast cancer mortality correlates more strongly with the consumption of milk-fat than with other types of fat. The enzyme Lactase, which is needed for milk-fat digestion, is thought to be implicated in the malignant change. Whole milk is a high-calorie food which presents grave disadvantages over skimmed milk. Whereas the protein, vitamin and carbohydrate content is identical in both, the fat content of skimmed milk is one twentieth that of whole milk which means that there are only 200 calories in one pint of skimmed milk, but 375, nearly *double*, in one pint of whole milk. This high-calorie content of whole milk is exclusively due to the presence of fat, a substance which, though pleasing to the palate, can be harmful to health.

Another factor affecting the breast is childbirth, in that the development of breast cancer in child-bearing women becomes progressively less likely as the age of the first pregnancy decreases. The earlier the first pregnancy, the less likely is the woman to suffer from breast cancer. This may be due to the effect of the first stimulus to lactation. This diminished risk is reinforced by a late onset of menstruation at puberty, particularly when this was due to under-nutrition: another example of the protective effect on health of dietary restriction. On the other hand over-nutrition and the resulting obesity increases the risk of both breast and uterine cancer.

9 STRESS

Emotional stress is a condition known to contribute to heart disease, high blood pressure, strokes and cancer. A human being is not merely a chemical factory or a primitive biological creature but an entity, comprising body, mind and spirit. It is the harmonious inter-relationship of these three components which determines one's state of well-being.

Stress has a debilitating effect on the body's immune system; though it is not the actual cause of the illness, it may be the determinant factor which swings the balance in a borderline condition. This is why certain illnesses cannot be explained in purely physical terms and why other factors such as anxiety, insecurity, emotional tension and stress play such an important part in their causation. Anxious people take much more out of themselves and thus become vulnerable to ill health. Nor is it unusual that the onset of illnesses such as cancer, a stroke or a coronary heart attack can be related to an emotional upset. Unless helped by counselling and meditation the troubled mind in such cases may continue to transmit its harmful messages to the body.

Unresolved problems, both real and imaginary, cause anxiety, and anxious people are tense and vulnerable. In other words they 'get stressed' and thus become more prone to disease. There is mounting evidence resulting from some recent work by neurobiologists, neurochemists and psychotherapists that mental stress can act as a precipitant of cancer. For instance the onset of cancer frequently relates to an emotional upset such as a bereavement, redundancy, retirement or a financial crisis etc. It is however not the actual personal grief or the severe blow which acts as the precipitant. It is the patient's reaction to it, or rather the lack of reaction to it, the bottling up, the failure to be able to communicate, which is the determinant. In other words it appears that the proneness to cancer relates to the patient's inability to express or discharge feelings. This is true to such an extent that it is possible, taking into account personality, to predict with a surprising degree of accuracy which individuals out of a group will eventually contract it. It seems that since suggestion, and in particular autosuggestion, transmits its messages to the body the mind is capable of altering the body's chemistry.

In summary, because negative emotions such as fear, anxiety, anger and jealousy can be as harmful to health as dietary excesses, one must deliberately eliminate them by voicing one's feelings freely to avoid the build-up of nervous tension which may lead to mental stress. For many, prayer and contemplation may be very effective by contributing to a more relaxed attitude of mind, but because the beneficial effects of meditation are still considered scientifically unproven, there are few reputable centres where this ancient method of mental relaxation is accepted as orthodox treatment. Other relaxation techniques which involve repeating a phrase or a prayer in comfortable quiet surroundings have been in use throughout the world for thousands of years and their beneficial effect, particularly in patients at risk from heart disease or high blood pressure, is irrefutable. This technique of 'mindless' prayer is thought to reduce excessive amounts of the hormone Noradrenaline which is produced under stress.

10 PHYSICAL EXERCISE

Regular exercise is one of the best ways of eliminating poisonous waste products that have accumulated in the body, thereby restoring the proper balance in the blood of its many essential constituents. Additionally, physical exercises tend to release pent-up emotions and thereby relieve mental stress.

There is ample evidence that lack of exercise contributes to the risk of atherosclerosis (hardening of the arteries), heart disease, hypertension (high blood pressure), strokes, obesity, diabetes and, last but not least, constipation.

The main purpose of exercise is to increase the efficiency of the heart and lungs, and it should be taken regularly, preferably for a period of 30–60 minutes at least five times per week — throughout an entire lifetime.

It is immaterial how exercise is taken; whether in the form of the 'daily dozen' or taking a long, brisk walk instead of driving the car or taking a bus; running upstairs two at a time rather than taking the lift; cycling long distances or energetically digging the garden. All these physical exertions in fit people should be gradually increased both in duration and vigour until a state of pronounced breathlessness and a marked increase in pulse rate is experienced at least once every day. However, even in extended vigorous exercises little of the massive energy contained in the dietary fat or sugar is used up; that is why there are so many unsuccessful overweight joggers who, unless they cut down on fats, sugar and alcohol, will always remain fat.

For the energetic business executive exercise is also the only reliable method of protection from the stresses of his or her life, particularly as these usually include heavy smoking and hard drinking as well as over-eating. In such cases, systematic physical exercise may well assume a life-saving role, when otherwise a heart attack or a stroke may be only a matter of time.

There is conclusive evidence that people fortunate enough to be able to engage in regular sporting activities are, as a result of the healthy exercise, usually in excellent mental and physical condition. They are generally relaxed and sleep well; they worry less and they have no desire to over-eat or smoke, neither do they crave alcohol. Not only is their blood pressure normal, their pulse rate is slow at rest, and, even more important, it increases only slightly on exertion.

Outdoor sports afford the added bonus of natural unfiltered sunlight which is essential for optimal body condition. Natural light affects the body's hormone system after entering the eyes through the pupils. This results in a general sense of well-being as well as an increase in efficiency and a decrease in fatigue and explains why natural sunlight has such a very significant association with a person's mood. Since the glass used for ordinary spectacles and contact lenses filters out ultraviolet light, these should be removed from time to time, or they should be made of special material which does not shield out ultraviolet light.

Physical exercise is better by far than any known drug or medicine because it cures more diseases, solves more problems and relieves more stress than any other single agent. In particular, by burning excess blood-fat for fuel and cleaning the arteries of their fatty deposits, it minimises the risk of atherosclerosis and, as already stated, prevents high blood pressure, strokes, heart disease, obesity, diabetes and gallstones — the disastrous consequences of stress, sloth and gluttony. One further important advantage of exercise is its stimulating effect on intestinal peristalsis which helps to prevent constipation and with it a host of complicating illnesses.

In short, the healthiest person is one who spends a lifetime in regular vigorous outdoor exercise. The best exercises are those demanding endurance. Basically, a sedentary person is sick and those who do not find time for exercise will later *have* to find time for sickness. Furthermore exercise promotes slimness because excess fat is lost through increased metabolic rate, which is boosted through physical exertion by up to 30 per cent.

As a result of regular exercise fat is eventually replaced by muscle, and since muscle tissue burns more calories per minute than fat tissue, a muscular body increases the 'idling speed' of our metabolism even further. In fact, exercise seems to be the only way permanently to lower the point at which the body weight tends to settle and dieting without exercise is unlikely to lower this 'set point'.

11 A DAILY ROUTINE FOR HEALTHY LIVING

Ideally you should plan to wake up at least 15 minutes before actually having to get up, to give the awakening mind time for serene contemplation as it proceeds to full wakefulness. This should be a smooth and gentle process which can be aided by soothing music but *not* by stressful radio news.

During this extra lie in, cat-like stretching movements of limbs and spine will loosen the joints after a night of immobility. Before getting out of bed you should sit up and slowly sip two glasses of water to help initiate a reflex-peristaltic wave through the intestines to expedite a regular early morning bowel action. Since about 65 per cent of the body is composed of water it is important to replenish the body's water reservoir by drinking at least four pints of water each day. It should always be drunk slowly while seated, not when standing up.

On rising from bed some simple gymnastic exercises will give further help to the muscles and joints that may have stiffened up overnight. These physical exercises should be followed by breathing exercises consisting of a dozen deep rhythmical inhalations and exhalations which will expand the lungs to the full. You should always breathe in through the nose but you may breathe out through either the nose or the mouth. Such breathing exercises should be repeated whenever convenient about every four hours throughout the day.

After exercising, you should proceed to the bathroom for a shower and a brisk rub down. Dental hygiene forms a most important part of health care, so the teeth should be thoroughly brushed (not forgetting to massage the gums) and this process should be repeated after each meal.

As regards clothing, remember that synthetic fibre like nylon is non-porous and does not allow the skin to breathe, so try to wear natural fibre such as cotton, wool or silk next to the skin. It is also important to avoid all constricting garments such as form-fitting jeans. It is better not to wear tight shoes and the heels should be neither too high nor too low, but just comfortable.

Allow at least half an hour for a leisurely breakfast and do not forget to brush your teeth again afterwards.

This very relaxed start, which is very important because it will set one up for the rest of the day, should be compared with the more usual, frenetic routine practices in the 'civilised' West, where a lightning catapult out of bed is followed by a quick dash to the bathroom, a hurried breakfast and a mad rush out of the house to the garage or to catch a train or bus.

Small wonder, then, after repeating this at least 300 times a year for 35 years, that many will have developed a high blood pressure and will eventually suffer a stroke, which after heart disease and cancer, is the third commonest cause of death.

The type of breakfast to be taken is a matter for individual preference but as a general guide: sugar, butter, cream, whole-milk products, fried eggs, fried bacon and white bread should be restricted whereas crude bran, whole-meal bread and fruit should always be included. It is not generally appreciated how very important it is to masticate well at all times.

It is also important to be always aware of one's posture and to try, consciously, to sit, stand or walk erect. This means upright, with the shoulders well back, the neck straight and the head held high. In this stance the head and the neck becomes a natural extension of the spine and this will prevent many of the painful ailments of the neck, shoulders, arms, back and legs in later life.

Instead of using transport all the way to work, at least part of the way should be covered on foot at a fairly brisk pace. This should include all stairs which should be welcomed as an ideal opportunity for sudden physical exertion. For those not going out to work, a vigorous morning walk or cycle ride is imperative before settling down to work at home and if this is of a sedentary nature then the morning's physical activities become absolutely mandatory.

During weekends, when staying at home, select the sport compatible with age, physical capacity and mental attitude, and never forget that walking is marvellous as a recreation.

Halfway through a working morning, perhaps during the coffee break, at least ten minutes should be spent in positive thinking: that is, in serene contemplation, which will re-charge the wearying mind. Before resuming work one should remember deep-breathing exercises and some simple gymnastic movements to relax the muscles and the joints of the spine. This will allow one to resume work refreshed and with renewed zest until lunch time.

A modest lunch is preferable, to be followed by a short brisk walk. During the subsequent rest period use the time for another session of serene contemplation followed by rhythmical deep breathing and light gymnastic movements.

Lunch is a matter of personal preference. Several small meals a day are better than one or two large ones. Yet again: sugar, butter, cream, whole-milk, cheeses, alcohol, fat meat, fried food, ice-creams, cakes and white bread are on the 'restricted items list', whilst wholemeal bread, baked or boiled potatoes, vegetables, fruit, fish and poultry are permitted.

Again, part of the homeward journey should be covered on foot. On arrival at home one should ensure a period of light-hearted conversation and relaxation before the evening meal. The art of laughing and of being cheerful should be cultivated at this and all other times, and anger and contention should be avoided. if possible one's philosophy should always be: 'Accept with grace what cannot be changed and try to be content with what you have.'

Large dinners should be reserved for the odd festive occasion when there is something to celebrate. A heavy meal at night interferes with sound sleep; in any case every large meal enhances the risk of obesity particularly when the food eaten is rich in sugar, fats and alcohol. The diet should always be balanced with the main emphasis being on proteins and roughage, that is on food rich in dietary fibre such as bran, wholemeal flour products, vegetables and fruit. In fact, roughage should proportionally form the largest single item in every meal and this important rule should be always adhered to.

And so to bed. A bedroom should be cool, unheated and airy. One should refrain from taking stimulants such as strong tea, coffee or alcohol after 5pm. To avoid a 'bad back', the mattress should be very firm, if not hard, as this promotes sound dreamless sleep and increases the likelihood of waking well rested and in a happy frame of mind.

Whereas 10 hours of sleep are permissible at the age of 20, with advancing years there is a gradually decreasing need for sleep and it is advisable to reduce the time spent in bed. Fit people need only 6–7 hours of sleep.

Conversely, from 20 years and on, it is really important to interrupt one's activities in the middle of the day for a brief rest-period with the feet up, eyes closed and complete mental relaxation. This 'cat-nap' is an invaluable asset and very important to cultivate. A 10 minutes rest at the age of 30 should be gradually increased to roughly 20 minutes at the age of 60.

Since natural unfiltered light is essential for optimal body conditions and ordinary spectacles and contact lenses shield out the ultraviolet rays, glasses or contact lenses should be removed for about ten minutes 2–3 times each day.

Part Two

RECIPES

INTRODUCTION

The main aim of this simple food guide is to make 'sensible eating' more tempting and less difficult, by listing a wide selection of specially thought out, simple recipes for tasty wholefood dishes that are inexpensive and easy to prepare. They are cooked with virtually no fat, sugar or salt, which makes then non-fattening; at the same time they are planned to contain, per calorie consumed, a very high fibre, protein, vitamin and mineral percentage, which makes them extremely nutritious. It is this rare dietary combination of being simultaneously low-calorie, fibre-rich and nutritious yet still mouth-watering that makes them such an ideal health food for everyone.

Since it is what we eat during our lifetime that influences the probability of developing cancer (as well as heart disease, high blood pressure, strokes and diabetes), the single most effective way of reducing this probability is to eat sensibly.

The Rules of Sensible Eating

1) Choose food low in fat, sugar and salt, but rich in fibre, protein, vitamins and minerals.

2) Cut down on butter, margarine, oil and cooking fats, as well as on whole milk, cream and cheese.

3) Reduce the consumption of eggs, red meat, processed and salty foods, sweet desserts and alcohol.

4) Replace white bread with wholemeal bread; exchange white flour products for wholemeal flour products; and swap puddings for fruit.

5) Prefer boiled or baked potatoes to chips; prefer grilled or steamed food to fried foods; and prefer porridge or muesli to eggs and bacon.

6) Adopt fruit, vegetables and whole-grain cereals as everyday staple diet in preference to meat, fats and confectionery.

7) Accept that cold food is not less nutritious than hot food; and that bread and potatoes are not more fattening than meat and fats.

8) Restrict the total daily amount of your food intake sufficiently not to cause obesity.

9) Always be painstakingly discriminating in your choice of food, even when invited out.

10) Subscribe joyfully to a new, more disciplined and thereby much safer way of life.

Substitutes

Since the most commonly consumed fats such as butter, margarine, cooking fats and oil are not only unnecessary but can actually be harmful, particularly when eaten regularly, fats have been left out of the recipes and replaced, where necessary, by skimmed milk soft cheese. Ideally, fish, poultry or veal should not be fried; they should be grilled, or cooked in stock and the excess fat skimmed off. When grilling, the food is brushed with stock, in place of fat. Even better, when first wrapped in foil it does not need to be brushed and, besides, it retains all its moisture, flavour and goodness.

Since sugar (whether taken as white sugar, brown sugar, raw sugar, Demerara sugar, molasses, syrup or honey) is extremely fattening and totally without nutritional value, it is not used in the recipes; in its place, harmless, low-calorie, artificial sweeteners are used. Whether liquid or in tablet form, sweeteners are very concentrated and are best and most exactly used when first diluted in water. The more water is used for the dilution the easier it is to get the taste exactly right. When in tablet form, dissolve in a tablespoon or larger quantity of boiling water in a cup and then spoon out the required amount. Drops of sweetener should be similarly diluted with a tablespoon, or more, of cold water in a cup and then spooned out to taste.

As salt may contribute directly to high blood pressure and so to heart disease or a stroke and as it is difficult to determine in advance who is and who is not sensitive to salt and hypertension, it is best to reduce the salt intake for everyone. (Since calcium has been shown to reduce blood pressure, drinking at least one pint of skimmed milk a day is as important as avoiding salt.)

Three salt substitutes have been used to replace the sodium-rich, and thus potentially harmful, common salt in the recipes.

1) The diet-salt Ruthmol, unlike table-salt or sea-salt, is low in sodium-content and rich in potassium instead.

2) Miso, a flavouring substance, produced by cereal fermentation, is

rich in protein, vitamins and minerals.

3) Vecon is a yeast, iron and vitamin B12-containing vegetable concentrate.

Worthwhile foods

1) *High in protein-content*
Foods rich in high quality proteins and thus essential for maintenance of health, include fish, turkey, crab, lobster, chicken, veal, egg-white, yoghurt, skimmed milk, cottage cheese, beans, peas, Tofu (a defatted, low-calorie soya-bean curd), or Bipro (a pure protein extract).

2) *Rich in vitamins and minerals*
Essential vitamin-and-mineral-rich foods include carrots, cauliflower, Brussel sprouts, spinach, turnips, parsley, green peppers, watercress, broccoli, spinach and radishes.

3) *Rich in fibre*
bran, whole cereals, whole potatoes and whole fruit.
It should be noted that fruit and vegetables maintain a higher vitamin content if cooked by steaming lightly; better still, eat them raw.

Snacks and Treats

The temptation to eat between meals is often irresistible. To satisfy this ever-recurring craving, there should always be a bowl ready in the kitchen, or in the fridge, containing already cleaned raw snacks, handily sliced into holdable sticks of carrots, cauliflower, celery, courgettes, unshelled peas (which are great to pop), cucumber sticks or even an occasional whole tomato, or a lettuce leaf filled with a slice of courgette or cucumber and sprinkled, for more flavour, with a little diet-salt.

Alternatively a bowl of only-very-slightly-cooked (so that they are still crunchy) beans, broccoli, cauliflower, spinach or other green vegetables, quickly boiled in a little diet-salted water, represent a welcome change from the raw vegetable sticks.

At coffee-time or tea-time a slice of bran-crispbread (85 per cent bran) garnished either by a lettuce leaf and topped by a teaspoon of cottage cheese, or by a sliver of lean ham with a slice of tomato or cucumber and flavoured by diet-salt, are very acceptable. If, to keep happy, it has to be a sweet snack, the answer lies in either whole earth jams (containing no added sugar) or a squashed ripe fruit mashed up with a drop of liquid sweetener, on a piece of crispbread or wholemeal bread.

Additionally, if the craving for something sweet is compulsive then a small, strictly controlled amount of high-calorie confectionery (about 300 calories) is legitimately allowable as a reward for having religiously kept to a low-calorie, fibre-rich diet all day.

What to restrict to small amounts	What to eat regularly and plentifully
Butter	Bran
Cream	Unrefined cereals
Fatty meats	Wholemeal bread
Fried food	Whole wheat flour
Unskimmed milk	Unpolished rice
High fat cheeses	Vegetables
Mayonnaise	Fruit
Ice cream	Fish
Sugar and salt	Poultry
Confectionery	Skimmed milk
Alcohol	Low fat cheeses

Notes on the Recipes

The following recipes are from the Slimline Diet Kitchen of the Clinic for Cancer Prevention Advice run by Dr Jan de Winter in Brighton, England*, and were compiled by Daniele de Winter and Joanna C. Read.

They are divided up into the following categories: starters, soups, sandwiches, main courses, baked potatoes, salads and salad dressings, desserts, and biscuits and cakes. A guide to the number of calories in each serving is included in each recipe. 'Sauté' means to heat a small quantity of chicken or vegetable stock (not oil or fat) in a saucepan, and to add the food when simmering and brown quickly. 'Blanch' means to bring food rapidly to boiling point in water and boil for a very short time.

*6 New Road; telephone 0273 727213.

STARTERS

Melon

Serves 2–4

1 medium Melon, any variety
The juice from 1 lemon
Artificial sweetener to taste

1. Halve the melon, remove the pips and spoon the flesh into a large bowl.
2. Sprinkle with the lemon juice and sweetener and mix well. Chill before serving.

Approx. calories per serving: 15

Avocado and Tomato Cocktail

Serves 4

2 avocados (diced)
4 medium tomatoes (diced)

Dressing
4 tablespoons vinegar
Low sodium salt and pepper
2 tablespoons yoghurt
1 teaspoon mild English mustard
1 tablespoon water
A few drops sweetener

1. First mix avocados and tomatoes.
2. Then mix dressing (start with yoghurt and mustard then add vinegar). Pour over vegetables and serve with wholemeal toast.

Approx. calories per serving: 171

Avocado with Shrimps

Serves 4

2 avocados
225 g (½ lb) shrimps
150 g (5 fl oz/¾c) natural yoghurt
1 flat tablespoon tomato puree
Juice from half a lemon
1 tablespoon vinegar
Low sodium salt
Pepper
Some finely cut lettuce
2 drops sweetener if desired

1. Halve avocados, remove stone and divide shrimps and lettuce between the 4 halves.
2. Cream vinegar with tomato puree, stir into yoghurt and add low sodium salt, pepper, lemon juice and sweetener to taste.
3. Pour over shrimps and serve with wholemeal bread.

Approx. calories per serving: 230

Globe Artichokes

Serves 4

4 globe artichokes
2 teaspoons finely chopped fresh sage
3 tablespoons concentrated vegetable stock
100 g (4 fl oz) low fat yoghurt
100g (4 oz/½c) skimmed milk cottage cheese
Low sodium salt
Pepper

1. Prepare artichokes. Break off the tough leaves and stem and trim the points off all leaves. Place in a pan of boiling low sodium salted water and simmer for 30–40 minutes. Drain, turn the artichokes upside down to dry and cool. Then remove small spiky inner leaves and choke — replace choke afterwards — stand artichokes in a serving dish.
2. Cream yoghurt and cottage cheese in a small pan and heat *very* gently and do not allow to boil. Stir in the vegetable stock and sage and when hot,

remove from heat. Season with low sodium salt and pepper and pour into each artichoke.

3. Serve remainder in a sauce-boat with artichokes.

Approx. calories per serving: 100

Smoked Herring/Mackerel Paté

Serves 4

250 g (9 oz/1c) low fat cottage cheese
1 large smoked herring (mackerel)
1 black olive, finely chopped
Lemon juice and pepper
1 teaspoon finely chopped parsley

1. Remove fish from bone and mash with a fork. Cream with cottage cheese and mix in chopped olive, a little lemon juice and the chopped parsley.

2. Season with salt and pepper, and serve on a bed of lettuce with wholemeal toast.

Approx. calories per serving: 157

SOUPS

Thick Chunky Vegetable Soup

Serves 6–8

1 large onion
2 carrots
1 large potato
1 turnip or swede (medium)
2 sticks of celery
2 leeks
½ small cauliflower
4 tomatoes
1 clove garlic crushed
1200 ml (2 pts/5c) vegetable stock (cube or homemade)
2 teaspoons chopped fresh mixed herbs
(or 1 teaspoon dried herbs)
50 g (2 oz) wholewheat macaroni
50 g (2 oz) frozen peas
Low sodium salt
Pepper

1. Wash and cube onion, carrots, potato, turnip; slice celery and leeks; break up cauliflower; skin and cube tomatoes.
2. Gently heat onion and garlic in a large pan for 2 minutes with 4 tablespoons of stock. Add celery, carrot and turnip, stirring for 5 minutes. Add remaining stock, herbs and tomatoes. Bring to the boil, then lower heat and simmer for 20 minutes. Stir in potatoes, leeks, cauliflower and macaroni and cook for 15–20 minutes. 5 minutes before end add peas and season with low sodium salt and pepper (add more stock if necessary).
3. Serve with wholemeal rolls or wholemeal croutons on soup, and if desired, a small pot of cottage cheese with chives.

Approx. calories per serving: 60

Tomato Soup and Tofu

Serves 4

450 g (1 lb) tomatoes (diced)
1 onion (chopped)
1 clove garlic (crushed)
2 teaspoons chopped fresh basil (1 teaspoon dried)
750 ml (1¼ pt/3c) vegetable stock
150 ml (¼ pt/½c) skimmed milk
3 tablespoons tomato puree
280 g (10 oz) Tofu (diced)
Low sodium salt
Pepper
Chopped fresh parsley
A blob of plain yoghurt as garnish

1. Heat onion and garlic in 4 tablespoons vegetable stock, in a pan for a few minutes. Add diced tomatoes and basil, continue cooking for a few minutes then stir in vegetable stock, tomato puree and milk. Bring to the boil, reduce heat and simmer for 15–20 minutes.
2. Remove from heat, add diced Tofu and pass mixture through blender. Season with low sodium salt and pepper (add some more stock or milk if too thick).
3. Return to pan and heat gently.
4. Serve with a blob of yoghurt, parsley and wholemeal croutons if desired.

Approx. calories per serving: 95

Watercress Soup

Serves 4

1 large onion (chopped)
1 clove garlic (crushed)
1 large bunch watercress (chopped)
225 g (8 oz) potatoes (finely sliced — unpeeled)
900 ml (1½ pts/3¾c) vegetable stock
140 ml (5 fl oz/¾c) plain yoghurt
Low sodium salt, pepper and paprika
(Few sprigs of watercress for garnish)
1 tablespoon Miso

1. Gently sauté onion and garlic in 4 tablespoons vegetable stock, in a large pan for 5 minutes. Add chopped watercress and continue cooking for 5 minutes. Add potatoes. Cook for 3–5 minutes and then add remaining stock, bring to boil and simmer until potatoes are soft (10 minutes).
2. Remove pan from heat and stir in yoghurt. Pass mixture through a sieve. Return mixture to pan and heat gently (do not boil).
3. Combine the Miso with a little of the soup until it is a paste, then stir into the soup.
4. Season, serve garnished with watercress and a little paprika.

Approx. calories per serving: 85

Cucumber Dill Soup

Serves 4

2 cucumbers (thinly sliced)
1 big bunch dill (chopped)
600 ml (1 pt/2½c) vegetable stock
1 onion (diced)
140 ml (5 fl oz/¾c) natural yoghurt
Low sodium salt
Pepper
Grated nutmeg
1 clove garlic
A little paprika
1 teaspoon Vecon

1. Heat onion in 3 tablespoons stock in a pan for a few minutes. Add cucumber and garlic and cook for another 5 minutes. Add dill and stock, and bring to boil. Reduce heat and simmer for 15 minutes.
2. Remove from heat, pass through blender and return to pan. On low heat, add yoghurt, salt and pepper, nutmeg and paprika and Vecon to taste. Do not allow yoghurt to boil.
3. Serve garnished with a little paprika.

Approx. calories per serving: 47

Cold Parsnip Soup

Serves 4

2 leeks (sliced)
2 sticks celery (sliced)
4 medium parsnips (diced)
100 g (4 oz) peas
900 ml (1½ pts/3¾c) vegetable stock
Low sodium salt
Pepper
300 ml (½ pt/1c) milk (skimmed)
Chopped fresh chives to garnish

1. Heat leeks and celery (without oil) in pan for a few minutes with 4 tablespoons of stock. Then add diced parsnips, peas, remaining stock, low sodium salt and pepper. Bring to the boil, then lower heat and simmer for 10–15 minutes (until parsnips are soft).
2. When vegetables are slightly cooled, pass them through a sieve or liquidizer, stir in milk, adjust seasoning and chill for 2–3 hours. (Alternatively try hot.)
3. Serve with chives.

Approx. calories per serving: 80

Gazpacho

Serves 4

500 ml (1 pt/2½c) tomato juice
½ cucumber (diced)
1 green pepper (diced)
1 onion (smallish — diced)
4 tomatoes (diced)
1 clove garlic (crushed)
Plenty of low sodium salt and pepper (soy sauce if desired)
1 tablespoon fresh chopped basil
1 tablespoon fresh chopped parsley
1 tablespoon fresh chopped dill

1. Put tomato juice into blender. Put aside half of the diced, chopped

cucumber, pepper and tomato and place the rest in blender along with onion and crushed garlic. Add low sodium salt and pepper, 3 tablespoons vinegar and ½ teacup skimmed milk. Blend and add basil, parsley and dill and chill for 2 hours (if too thick, add a few ice cubes).

2. Serve garnished with diced vegetables and wholemeal toast.

Approx. calories per serving: 57

Chilled Fruit Soup

Serves 4–6

450 g (1 lb) strawberries
2 large dessert apples
1 litre (1 ¾ pts/4½c) fruit juice (orange/apple)
20–30 drops liquid saccharin (or 6 tablets dissolved/crushed)
2 tablespoons cornflour
140 ml (5 fl oz/1 ¾c) natural yoghurt

1. Put aside 4 strawberries for garnishing. Press through sieve.
2. Peel, core and finely grate apples; put all fruit with sweetener and all but 4 tablespoons of fruit juice into a pan. Bring to boil, reduce heat and simmer for a few minutes. Whisk the cornflour into the remainder of the fruit juice and add to pan for another 10 minutes stirring continuously. Remove from heat, allow to cool and chill before serving.
3. Serve in bowls garnished with a spoonful of yoghurt and a strawberry.

Approx. calories per serving: 116

SANDWICHES

Serves 1

Tomato and Asparagus
2 slices wholemeal bread
1 tomato (sliced)
2 asparagus stalks (sliced)
1 tablespoon cottage cheese
Low sodium salt and pepper

Approx. calories per filling: 58

Chicken
2 slices wholemeal bread
50 g (2 oz) thinly sliced chicken
1 tablespoon cottage cheese
1 sliced tomato
4 lettuce leaves
Low sodium salt and pepper

Approx. calories per filling: 115

Shrimp
2 slices wholemeal bread
2 tablespoons peeled shrimps/prawns
1 tablespoon sensible 1,000 island dressing
4 thin cucumber slices
4 small lettuce leaves

Approx. calories per filling: 70

Alternative fillings
1. ½ mashed Avocado with 1 tablespoon yoghurt and a little lemon juice
on a bed of lettuce sprinkled with salt.

2. Any left-over boiled vegetables with a little cottage cheese, lettuce and sliced chicken meat (optional).

3. Any ripe, fresh fruit simply mashed on its own (apricots, peaches, strawberries) or with sweetener and lemon juice and (if desired) a little plain yoghurt.

Bread: Approx. calories per slice: 70

MAIN COURSES

Nutty Baked Vegetables

Serves 4

2 large sliced onions
2 sliced leeks
2 large sliced carrots
½ small chopped cabbage
2 teaspoons fresh thyme — chopped
Dash of soya sauce
Low sodium salt — salt substitute
Pepper
75 g (3 oz) coarsely chopped roasted peanuts
75 g (3 oz) dried wholemeal breadcrumbs

1. Sauté the onions in a large pan with a little stock for 5 minutes. Add the carrots and after 5 more minutes cooking add the leeks and cabbage, simmering for another 5 minutes. Remove from heat. (N.B. Vegetables should be tender but crunchy. If you prefer them cooked through, spinkle them with water and simmer for another 5 minutes until soft.)
2. Transfer the vegetables to a shallow oven proof dish and sprinkle in the thyme, soya sauce, low sodium salt and pepper to taste. Mix the peanuts and breadcrumbs together and sprinkle evenly over the vegetables. Bake for about 20 minutes — oven 180°C/350°F/Gas 4 — and garnish with a spoonful of cottage cheese if desired.

Approx. calories per serving: 190

Vegetable Rice

Serves 4–6

250 g (10 oz) brown rice
25 g (1 oz) peanuts (optional)
4 medium chopped tomatoes
1 large Spanish onion, sliced thin
2 medium sliced courgettes
2 medium thickly sliced leeks
½ cauliflower, broken into florets
3 tablespoons chopped fresh herbs
2 tablespoons chopped fresh parsley
1 crushed garlic clove
A pinch saffron
A pinch nutmeg
Low sodium salt
Pepper
Vegetable or chicken stock*
25 g (1 oz) raisins
3 teaspoons Vecon, to taste

*To check the relationship of rice to stock, when poured into a jug there must be 1½ times as much liquid as uncooked rice.

1. Put the onion and garlic, with 3–5 tablespoons of the measured stock, into the base of a large pressure cooker and steam gently for 5 minutes. Add the rice, courgettes, leeks, cauliflower, tomatoes, half the herbs and parsley, the nutmeg and saffron and the peanuts and stir well for 2 minutes.
2. Pour all the stock onto the mixture and close the pressure cooker. Bring to the boil on a high heat and as soon as the cooker begins to hiss, reduce the heat and simmer. Pressure cook for 20 minutes, and then reduce pressure and open. Check that there is still enough liquid, add the remaining herbs and season with low sodium salt, pepper; stir Vecon and raisins into the rice. Close and pressure cook for another 15 minutes or until rice is cooked.
3. Serve with a large mixed salad.

Approx. calories per serving: 225

Moussaka

Serves 4

170 g (6 oz) soya mince
56 g (2 oz) millet
35 ml (12 fl oz/1¼c) water
2 large thinly sliced aubergines
2 large sliced onions
140 ml (¼ pt/½c) concentrated vegetable stock
2 teaspoons dried mixed herbs
4 large sliced tomatoes
2 tablespoons tomato puree
140 ml (5 fl oz/¾c) low fat plain yoghurt
2 medium sliced courgettes
4 tablespoons skimmed milk
½ green pepper cut in cubes
Pepper
Cayenne pepper
½ tablespoon Vecon
Parsley sprigs to garnish

1. Put the soya mince in a pan with the water and bring to the boil. Lower the heat and simmer gently for 5 minutes. Drain, but keep the liquid.
2. Put the millet in a small pan and just cover with some of the hot soya liquid. Bring to the boil and simmer for 15 minutes. Drain, but keep the liquid.
3. Now put 2 tablespoons of the stock in a pan and lightly sauté the aubergine slices for 5 minutes, turning once. Remove them and repeat the process with the green peppers, courgettes and a little more stock. Drain and remove from the pan. Sauté the onions and tomatoes for 2 minutes in some stock, add the soya mince and cook gently for a few minutes. Season generously with half the herbs, and both types of pepper.
4. Arrange the mince mixture in a medium ovenproof dish, top with aubergines and the remainder of the herbs, then add the courgettes and lastly, the millet. Stir together the remainder of the vegetable stock with the tomato puree and pour over the whole dish. Cover the casserole and bake in the oven for 20 minutes — 180°C/350°F/Gas 4.

Beat the yoghurt, milk and cayenne pepper, take the casserole from the oven and pour in the mixture and bake — uncovered — for a further 30 minutes. Serve hot, garnished with parsley.

Moussaka goes well with millet and a mixed salad of tomatoes, a variety of greens, onions, cucumber, etc.

Approx. calories per serving: 274

Mixed Grain Pilau

Serves 4

2 chopped onions
1 chopped red pepper
1 crushed clove garlic
1 teaspoon ground cumin
½ teaspoon ground coriander
2 bay leaves
225 g (8 oz) mixed cooked grains (rice, wholewheat grains, kasha, millet)
100 g (4 oz) cooked peas
50 g (2 oz) sultanas, or less if desired
Low sodium salt — salt substitute
Pepper
2 hard boiled eggs
50 g (2 oz) cooked chopped soya beans
Paprika

1. Heat the chopped onion, red pepper and garlic in 4 tablespoons water for a few minutes. Add the spices and bay leaf and cook for a further 1 to 2 minutes.
2. Stir in the grains, peas and sultanas, mix well and continue cooking gently for 20-25 minutes until the grains are cooked.
3. Chop the eggs coarsely and season with a little low sodium salt, pepper and paprika and mix with the chopped soya beans. Sprinkle over the pilau.

Approx. calories per serving: 350

Jacket Parsnips

Serves 2

4 medium parsnips with tops removed
75 g (3 oz) ham-flavoured soya chunks
175 g (6 fl oz/½c) water
1 large chopped onion
50 g (2 oz) canned sweetcorn
Low sodium salt — salt substitute
Pepper
Chopped fresh parsley

1. Scrub the skins and chop the long, thin ends off the parsnips so that they

stand firm. Stand them on a baking sheet and bake for about 1 hour until tender. Oven 190°C/375°F/Gas 5.

2. While the parsnips are cooking, prepare the filling.

3. Put the soya chunks in a pan with the water, bring to the boil and simmer for 20–30 minutes. (Follow the instructions on the packet.)

4. Drain and leave on one side.

5. Heat the onion in a pan with a little water and after 5 minutes add the soya chunks while stirring. After another 5 mintues add the drained sweetcorn and heat through. Season with low sodium salt and pepper.

6. When the parsnips are soft, place two on each plate and pile the filling on top, garnishing with chopped parsley.

Approx. calories per serving: 250

Lentil Stuffed Courgettes

Serves 3–4

6 medium courgettes
1 diced onion
2 diced tomatoes
2 finely sliced sticks of celery
100 g (4 oz) red split lentils
2 teaspoons chopped fresh mixed herbs
50 g (2 oz) grated cheddar cheese
Low sodium salt — salt substitute
Pepper

1. Parboil the courgettes in salted boiling water for 2–3 minutes. Drain well, cut lengthways and scoop out and chop the flesh. Put the onion, tomatoes and celery into a pan and sauté for a few minutes. Add the lentils and enough water to cover, and simmer for about 20 minutes until all the water has been absorbed. Sprinkle with herbs and season with low sodium salt substitute and pepper.

2. Fill the courgette skins with the mixture and place side by side on thinly greased cooking foil in a dish. Sprinkle with cheese and grill for 5–10 minutes. Serve with French beans or spinach.

Approx. calories per serving: 170

Courgettes Provençale

Serves 4–6

175 g (6 oz) haricot beans soaked in water overnight
1 sliced green pepper
1 sliced onion
1 crushed garlic clove
225 g (8 oz) thickly cubed tomatoes
450 g (1 lb) courgettes
Low sodium salt — salt substitute
Pepper
1–2 teaspoons crushed dried rosemary
140 ml (5 fl oz/¾c) natural yoghurt

1. Drain the beans and cook in fresh boiling water for about 45 minutes until tender. Drain and leave on one side.
2. Sauté the onion, peppers and garlic in a little stock for 5 minutes. Add the tomato cubes and after a few minutes, add the courgettes. Sprinkle with rosemary, low sodium salt and pepper, stir well and simmer for 10–15 minutes, and then stir in the beans and heat through.
3. Transfer the vegetables onto a serving dish and spoon the yoghurt over. Serve with wholemeal rice and a green salad.

Approx. calories per serving: 108

Winter Vegetable Stew

Serves 4

1 large diced turnip
1 large diced parsnip
2 sliced carrots
2 sliced leeks
¼ large shredded cabbage
1 sliced onion
75 g (3 oz) pearl barley or pot barley (soaked in water overnight and drained)
1 teaspoon fresh chopped thyme
1 teaspoon Miso
Low sodium salt — salt substitute
Pepper
About 1.15 litres (2 pts/5c) chicken stock (2 cubes)

1. Put all the prepared ingredients except the Miso into a large saucepan. Season with a little low sodium salt and pepper and pour in just enough stock to cover.
2. Bring to the boil, cover and simmer gently over a low heat for one to one and a half hours (2–3 hours when using hot barley) until the grain is tender.
3. Dilute Miso with a little hot water. Add to the stew and cook for one more minute. Serve with warm wholemeal rolls and a green salad.

Approx. calories per serving: 150

Hot Stuffed Tomatoes

Serves 2–3

4 large tomatoes
50 g (2 oz) mushrooms
1 clove garlic (crushed)
100 g (4 oz) cooked brown rice
2 tablespoons chopped parsley and basil
75 g (3 oz) cottage cheese
Low sodium salt and pepper
1 tablespoon tomato puree
2 tablespoons skimmed milk

1. Wash and dry tomatoes, cut a slice from the round end of each one and scoop out inside — chop coarsely. Sauté mushrooms in 2 tablespoons milk with a third of the cottage cheese and garlic until soft (3–5 minutes). Stir in cooked rice, tomato pulp, tomato puree, herbs, salt and pepper and the remainder of the cottage cheese and mix well.
2. Divide the filling between the tomatoes and put on tomato lids. Arrange in a shallow ovenproof dish and bake for 10–15 minuts (until puffed up) — oven 190°C/375°F/Gas 5. Serve hot or cold. (Serve cold with baked potato and mixed salad — serve hot with brown rice and boiled/steamed French beans or steamed courgettes. Hot or cold, serve with hot tomato sauce.)

Approx. calories per serving: 184

Tomato Sauce

Serves 2

1 onion (chopped)
2 cloves garlic (crushed)
4 tomatoes (chopped)
3 tablespoons tomato puree
70 ml (2.5 fl oz/ ⅜ c) natural yoghurt
Low sodium salt and pepper
Artificial sweetener to taste
Chopped chives

1. Put all ingredients into liquidizer and blend, season to taste with sweetex, low sodium salt and pepper. Pour into a pan and heat gently, not allowing to boil. Transfer to a gravy boat and top with plenty of chopped olives.

Approx. calories per serving: 75

Sweet Corn Ratatouille

Serves 4

1 large diced aubergine
1 large sliced green or red pepper
1 large sliced onion
2 thickly sliced courgettes
3 large chopped tomatoes
1 crushed garlic clove
100 g (4 oz) canned sweetcorn
2 bay leaves
Low sodium salt — salt substitute
Pepper
25 g (1 oz) walnut pieces
1 level teaspoon chopped fresh rosemary

1. Sprinkle the diced aubergine with salt and set aside for 30 minutes.
2. In ⅛ pt (¼c) stock heat the onion, garlic and pepper slices and simmer gently, stirring frequently for 5 minutes. Rinse and pat dry the aubergine pieces and together with the courgettes and the chopped rosemary add to the pan. Cook for another 10 minutes.

3. Now add the tomatoes, drained sweetcorn, bay leaves and low sodium salt and pepper to taste. Cover the pan and simmer for about 10 minutes until the vegetables are just cooked.

4. Remove the bay leaf. Stir in the walnut pieces, season to taste with low sodium salt and pepper and sherbs such as thyme or chives.

5. Sprinkle with parsley and serve with baked jacket potatoes, wholemeal pasta, brown rice or millet.

Approx. calories per serving: 112

Cauliflower Cheese

Serves 4

1 large cauliflower
175 g (6 oz/¾c) cottage cheese
140 ml (5 fl oz/¾c) plain yoghurt
1 tablespoon wholemeal flour
25–50 g (1–2 oz/¼c) wholemeal breadcrumbs
1 teaspoon chopped fresh mixed herbs
Low sodium salt — salt substitute
Pepper
5 tablespoons skimmed milk
2 teaspoons Vecon

1. Break the cauliflower into florets and cook in boiling salted water for 5–10 minutes. Drain and arrange in a shallow ovenproof dish.

2. Stir together the cottage cheese, yoghurt, flour, breadcrumbs, herbs and skimmed milk. Season with low sodium salt and pepper and spoon the mixture over the cauliflower. Bake for about 10 minutes in a moderate oven — 180°C/350°F/Gas 4.

3. Serve with wholegrain rice and a mixed salad.

4. Broccoli, courgettes, leeks spinach and most other vegetables may be prepared in exactly the same way.

Approx. calories: 200 per large portion
130 per average portion

Cauliflower with Pasta

Serves 4

1 medium cauliflower (broken into florets)
350 g (12 oz) wholewheat pasta shells
1 clove garlic (crushed)
300 ml (½ pt/1c) tomato sauce* (*see tomato sauce)
Salt and pepper
12 green olives and
1 tablespoon chopped fresh parsley as garnish

1. Boil or steam cauliflower florets in a little salted water for about 5 minutes until almost cooked and in a separate pan of salted boiling water, cook the pasta shells for 10 minutes until just tender.
2. Heat the garlic in a frying pan in a little water and immediately add tomato sauce, low sodium salt and pepper to taste. Heat through.
3. Drain pasta and cauliflower and mix them together in a serving dish. Pour the sauce over the top and garnish with olives and parsley.
Alternative: Instead of the tomato sauce, a cucumber and dill sauce, basil sauce or cottage cheese and chive sauce can be used. Blanched courgettes, broccoli or white cabbage can be used instead of the cauliflower.

Approx. calories per serving: 340

Spinach Lasagne

Serves 4–6

225 g (8 oz) wholewheat lasagne
225 g (8 oz) spinach
225 g (8 oz/1c) cottage cheese
1 beaten egg
1 crushed garlic clove
1 small onion
2 teaspoons chopped fresh basil
25 g (1 oz) parmesan cheese
Low sodium salt — salt substitute
Pepper
2 teaspoons Vecon
1 tablespoon natural yoghurt

1. Cook the lasagne in a pan of boiling salted water until soft (5 minutes for

home-made, 15 minutes for shop bought). Drain and rinse in cold water.

2. Wash and shred the spinach. Place in a wet pan; cover and steam very hot for 5–10 minutes until tender. Drain and mix with basil, onion and garlic.

3. Beat the cottage cheese, egg, Vecon and yoghurt and season with a little low sodium salt and pepper.

4. Arrange half the lasagne across the bottom of a shallow ovenproof casserole and cover with half the spinach and then half the cottage cheese mixture. Repeat this and sprinkle the top with parmesan.

5. Bake for 30 minutes until the top is well browned — oven 190°C/375°F/ Gas 5.

Approx. calories per serving: 208

Aubergine with Yoghurt

Serves 4

2 large sliced aubergine
2 sliced onions
2 crushed garlic cloves
150 g (1 lb) tomatoes
2 medium sliced courgettes
Low sodium salt
Pepper
½ teaspoon cayenne
1 teaspoon ground cumin
140 ml (5 fl oz/¾c) natural yoghurt
1 tablespoon tomato puree

1. Mix the tomato puree with three tablespoons of concentrated chicken stock and set aside. Lay the sliced aubergine on a plate and sprinkle with salt. Leave for half an hour and then rinse in cold water and pat dry with absorbent kitchen paper.

2. Put half the aubergine sliced in a shallow ovenproof dish. Heat the onion and garlic with the diluted tomato puree in a pan and after 5 minutes stir in the tomatoes, courgettes, spices, low sodium salt and pepper. Continue stirring for 5 minutes, then remove from heat and spread half the mixture over the aubergine, and repeat layer by layer — aubergine, tomato/ courgette mixture — and top with the yoghurt. Bake for 40–50 minutes — oven 180°C/350°F/Gas 4.

Approx. calories per serving: 105

Sweet Savoury Rice

Serves 6

3 sliced bananas
50 g (2 oz) peanuts
25 g (1 oz) cashew nuts
50 g (2 oz) sweetcorn, tinned and drained
25 g (1 oz) sultanas
A pinch of cinnamon
A few drops of artificial sweetener to taste
50 g (2 oz) sesame seeds
A pinch of low sodium salt — salt substitute
225 g (8 oz) brown rice
600 ml (1 pt/2½c) water
1 crushed garlic clove
2–3 tablespoons Miso
2 finely chopped onions
1 chopped green pepper
2 tablespoons dried mixed herbs

1. Put the rice and 4 tablespoons of water in the bottom of a large pressure cooker. Stir over a gentle heat until heated through and then add the nuts, sesame seeds, sultanas, cinnamon, herbs and low sodium salt. Stir well, add the water and seal the pressure cooker.
2. Bring to the boil and then lower the heat and simmer for 35–40 minutes. After 30 minutes simmering remove from heat and add the sweetcorn, sweetener and pepper and more water if necessary. Cook for another 10 minutes and add the sliced bananas.
3. Serve if desired, with a spoonful of plain yoghurt. Alternatively serve with a lettuce and apple salad with sweet vinegar dressing.

Approx. calories per serving: 315

Golden Carrot Quiche

Serves 4

Base
75 g (3 oz) wholemeal flour
25 g (1 oz) soya flour

50 g (2 oz/¼c) curd cheese
Cold water
Pinch of low sodium salt

1. Mix the curd cheese with the wholemeal and soya flours, rub the cheese
into the mixture until it resembles crumbs, then add cold water until a
dough is formed. Roll out and line a lightly greased medium sized flan dish.

Filling
100 g (4 oz) carrots (sliced)
50 g (2 oz/¼c) cottage cheese
100 g (4 oz/½c) curd cheeses
4 tablespoons natural low fat yoghurt
1 teaspoon ground nutmeg
Low sodium salt and pepper

1. Boil the carrots in water until they are soft. Mash them with the cottage
and curd cheeses, add the yoghurt, nutmeg, low sodium salt and pepper and
stir well.
2. Fill the case and bake for approximately 25 minutes until golden. Serve
with a green or a mixed salad.

Approx. calories per serving: 174

Sunflower Seed Burgers

Serves 4

100 g (4 oz) ground sunflower seeds
100 g (4 oz/½c) wholemeal breadcrumbs
2 teaspoons fresh chopped basil or 1 teaspoon dried chopped basil
1 teaspoon fresh chopped thyme
 Low sodium salt — salt substitute
Pepper
1 finely chopped spanish onion
1 crushed garlic clove
150 ml (¼ pt/½c) vegetable stock
50 g (2 oz) plain wholemeal flour

1. Put the sunflower seeds, breadcrumbs, herbs and little low sodium salt, a
little pepper, the onion and garlic in a bowl and mix well. Add the vegetable
stock and (saving a little stock for brushing the burgers) continue to mix

vigorously. Using floured hands, shape the mixture into 4–6 burgers, depending on the size. Stir some low sodium salt and pepper into the flour and dip each burger into the mixture to coat it thoroughly. Brush the burgers with some more vegetable stock and lay them on a very thinly oiled baking sheet and bake for 30 minutes turning them once — oven 180°C/350°F/Gas 4.

Approx. calories per serving: 250

Onion and Tomato Bake

Serves 4–6

275 g (10 oz) shelled broad beans
3 large sliced onions
450 g (1 lb) sliced tomatoes
3 tablespoons fresh basil — more if preferred (chopped)
1 crushed garlic clove
Low sodium salt — salt substitute
Pepper
50 g (2 oz/¼c) dried wholemeal breadcrumbs

1. Cook the broad beans in boiling salted water for about 20 minutes. Drain and leave on one side.
2. Gently heat the onions with 3 tbsp of stock in a pan until soft.
3. In the base of a shallow ovenproof dish arrange half the onion and cover with half the beans and top with half the tomatoes, half the basil and add low sodium salt and pepper. Repeat this and finally top with breadcrumbs. Bake for 20 minutes — oven 200°C/400°F/Gas 6.

Approx. calories per serving: 87

Onion and Tomato Bake with Fish

Serves 6

The ingredients are as above with the following additions:

275 g (10 oz) filleted plaice or sole
½ thinly sliced lemon

1. Heat the fillets with the onion, sprinkled with a little low sodium salt, pepper and basil. Arrange half the quantity in the base of the pan and cover with half the lemon slices. Repeat this and proceed as above.

Approx. calories per serving: 130

Vegetable Curry

Serves 4

2 chopped carrots*
1 chopped potato*
½ small cauliflower, in florets
2 sliced tomatoes*
50 g (2 oz) shelled fresh or frozen peas
100 g (4 oz) fresh or canned okra
1 finely chopped green pepper
1 finely chopped onion
1 teaspoon ground turmeric
2 teaspoons ground coriander
2 teaspoons ground cumin
1 teaspoon mustard seed
1 teaspoon curry powder
1 clove garlic, crushed
25 g (1 oz) cashew nuts, roasted
Low sodium salt — salt substitute
Pepper
50–75 g (2–3 oz) crushed sunflower seeds
140 ml (5 fl oz/¾c) natural yoghurt

*or about 675 g (1½ lb) vegetables of your choice.

1. Parboil the harder vegetables (peas, carrots, potatoes etc.) in salted boiling water for about 5 minutes. Drain and keep the water. In a large pan heat the onion, the garlic, green peppers and all the spices in two tablespoons of vegetable water, continually stirring for 5 minutes. Add all the vegetables to the pan, season with salt and pepper and pour in about half to one tea cup of the vegetable water. Cook gently for about 10 minutes until all the vegetables are tender but still crunchy (top up with water if necessary).
2. Sprinkle in crushed sunflower seed and nuts and cook for 5 minutes more, then add yoghurt and remove from heat.

73

3. Serve at once with plain boiled brown rice and a small side dish of sliced bananas, mango chutney, sliced cucumber in yoghurt and chopped peanuts and cashews.

Approx. calories per serving: 225

Soya or Chicken Curry

Serves 4

½ kg (1 lb) soya beef*
or ½ kg (1 lb) lean chicken, cubed
1 large finely chopped onion
2 crushed garlic cloves
1 heaped tablespoon Miso
570 ml (1 pt/2½c) chicken or beef stock
1 teaspoon madras curry powder
2 teaspoons madras chilli powder
1 tablespoon wholemeal flour
1 tablespoon pulverised sunflower seeds
3–4 drops sweetener

* The weight given on the pack when already hydrated; it weighs a lot less when dry.

1. Dissolve the Miso in hot water.
2. In the base of a pressure cooker, simmer chopped onion and garlic for five minutes with 4 tablespoons stock; then add the soya straight from the packet, *or* the chicken cubes, and heat, stirring for another five minutes.
3. Add the stock and stir in the curry and chilli powder and shut the pressure cooker. Cook over a medium to strong heat (almost boiling) for 30 minutes. Remove from heat, release the steam and open the pressure cooker.
4. Mix the sunflower seeds and sweetener with a little of the sauce and return to the curry; sprinkle in the flour and return to heat, stirring until the sauce thickens.
5. Serve with brown rice and a green salad — with bits of apple and onion if desired.

Approx. calories per serving: Soya Curry 380
Chicken Curry 235

74

Kebabs

Kebabs are best served with hot brown wholegrain rice spiced with turmeric (1 tablespoon turmeric sprinkled onto 450 g (1 lb) rice before cooking). Millet is also very acceptable — served with a generous sprinkling of chopped toasted pistachio nuts, or almonds. They can be made in many combinations, such as fruit and vegetable, vegetable and meat, or just vegetable alone. Here are 3 variations.

Fruit and Vegetable Kebab

Serves 4

2 thick slices toasted wholemeal bread, cut into cubes
1 large cubed parsnip
1 can 425 g (15½ oz) pineapple in natural juice
3 firm cubed bananas
3 thickly sliced courgettes
1 large cubed green pepper
100 g (4 oz) button mushrooms
350 g (12 oz) cherry tomatoes
Bay leaves
Low sodium salt — salt substitute
Pepper
140 ml (¼ pt/½c) vegetable stock

1. Prepare all the ingredients and thread them decoratively onto 12 skewers. Brush with stock and season with low sodium salt and pepper.
2. Lay the kebabs on a baking sheet and cook under a medium grill, turning frequently and brushing with stock. Great care must be taken to see that the fruit does not burn!
3. In about 10 minutes the kebabs should be well heated through. Serve immediately.

Approx. calories per serving: 200

Chicken Kebab

Serves 4

300 g (11 oz) chicken legs and/or breasts
1 cubed green pepper
100 g (4 oz) button mushrooms
350 g (12 oz) cherry tomatoes
2 medium onions cut into large cubes
3 medium sliced courgettes
1 teaspoon dried mixed herbs
Low sodium salt — salt substitute
Pepper
140 ml (¼ pt/½c) chicken stock
4 bay leaves

1. Remove the flesh from the bone and cut into cubes. Simmer for 10 minutes in the stock while the vegetables are prepared. Drain the chicken but keep the liquid. Assemble the ingredients onto 12 skewers placing chicken and vegetable alternately. Season with low sodium salt and pepper.
2. Cook exactly as the fruit and vegetable kebab for about 10 minutes, brushing the skewers frequently with stock.

Approx. calories per serving: 160

Fish Kebab

Serves 4

300 g (11 oz) diced cod, pike, carp or other similar fish
12 sardines

1. This dish is prepared in exactly the same way as chicken kebab, but add a tablespoon of lemon juice to the vegetable stock before simmering the cubed fish. (If vegetable stock is not available chicken stock will do very well.)

Approx. calories per serving: 225

Bean and Chicken Stew

Serves 6

350 g (12 oz) chicken meat
1 large onion, peeled and sliced
1 tablespoon wholemeal flour
280 ml (½ pt/1c) chicken stock
2 teaspoons tomato puree
1 teaspoon dried mixed herbs or 1 tablespoon fresh mixed herbs (chopped)
425 g (15 oz) red kidney beans
Low sodium salt — salt substitute
Pepper

1. Remove all skin and fat from the chicken and dice. Drain the kidney beans.
2. Steam the chicken and onion in ½ pt stock in a large saucepan for 5–10 minutes, then sprinkle on the flour and add the remainder of the stock. Bring to the boil, add the kidney beans, tomato puree and the herbs and stir well. Season to taste with low sodium salt and pepper, cover and simmer for ½–1 hour until the chicken is well cooked.
3. This dish is delicious when served with a boiled cauliflower (cooked in boiling water for 10 minutes), a tomato and onion salad and wholemeal bread.

Approx. calories per serving: 275

Tofu Chop Suey

Serves 4

1 chopped onion
1 chopped green pepper
¼ medium white cabbage, shredded
100 g (4 oz) sliced mushrooms
½ bunch of water cress
1 tablespoon arrowroot
1 tablespoon soya sauce (or more to taste)
5 to 10 drops of sweetener (dilute with water to facilitate measurement)
About 140 ml (¼ pt/½c) chicken stock
100 g (4 oz) coarsely chopped Tofu
100 g (4 oz) bean sprouts

1. Mix the arrowroot with the soya sauce, sweetener and the chicken stock in a small bowl.
2. Put the onion and green pepper in a large pan with a little water and heat gently for five minutes. Add the Tofu to the pan and mix well. Continue cooking for two more minutes, then add the cabbage, water cress and mushrooms and sauté for another two minutes, stirring frequently. Add the beansprouts and arrowroot solution and simmer all the ingredients until the sauce begins to thicken then add enough stock to make the sauce more liquid and heat through.
3. Serve with brown rice. (Soya sauce on the table.)

Approx. calories per serving: 70

Chicken Chop Suey

Serves 4

1 chopped onion
1 chopped green pepper
¼ medium white cabbage, shredded
100 g (4 oz) sliced mushrooms
½ bunch of water cress
1 tablespoon arrowroot
1 tablespoon soya sauce (or more to taste)
5 to 10 drops of sweetener (dilute with water to facilitate measurement)
About 140 ml (¼ pt/½c) chicken stock
200 g (8 oz) diced chicken meat
100 g (4 oz) bean sprouts

1. Mix the arrowroot with the soya sauce, sweetener and the chicken stock in a small bowl.
2. Put the onion and green pepper in a large pan with a little water and heat gently for five minutes. Add the chicken to the pan and mix well. Continue cooking for ten more minutes, then add the cabbage, water cress and mushrooms and sauté for another two minutes, stirring frequently. Add the beansprouts and arrowroot solution and simmer all the ingredients until the sauce begins to thicken then add enough stock to make the sauce more liquid and heat through.
3. Serve with brown rice (Soya sauce on the table).

Approx. calories per serving: 132

Paella

Serves 8–10

This is a delicious, very Spanish recipe. If mussels or lobster are not available, the dish will still be very good.

4 lobster claws, divided into several pieces
12 mussels
2 tablespoons finely chopped onion
4 tablespoons finely chopped parsley
140 ml (¼ pt/½c) chicken stock
1 chicken
225 g (8 oz) diced turkey
225 g (8 oz) ham-flavoured soya chunks
8 large whole prawns
1 large sliced courgette
1 large finely chopped Spanish onion
4 finely chopped garlic cloves
5 large peeled and chopped tomatoes
1 tin pimentos, cut in strips
Low sodium salt
Pepper, preferably fresh ground
¼ teaspoon cayenne pepper
½ teaspoon powdered saffron
570 ml (1 pt/2½c) chicken stock
450 g (1 lb) brown rice
1 tablespoon chopped fresh thyme

1. Remove all skin and fat from the chicken, take off the bone and dice. Bring the chicken stock to the boil.
2. Steam the mussels in ¼ pt chicken stock with 2 tablespoons each of onion, and parsley, until the shells open. Strain the mixture and keep the stock.
3. Steam the chicken and turkey pieces in the stock from the mussels (be sure the meat is covered) in a large covered saucepan for 15 minutes. Strain and keep the stock.
4. Steam the prawns and lobster if available in the same pan and the same stock for 5–10 minutes. Remove the prawns and lobster from the pan and steam the Spanish onion and 2 cloves of garlic until the onions are transparent. Add the tomatoes and pimentos and simmer for about 5 minutes, stirring constantly.
5. Return the steamed chicken, the turkey and *half* the mussels, prawns

and lobster to the pan, season with low sodium salt, pepper and Cayenne pepper and heat through.

6. Mix the remaining garlic, parsley, saffron and thyme in ¼ pt boiling stock, add to the remaining ¾ pt stock and pour over the meat mixture. Bring to the boil, stirring continuously and add the rice and courgettes.

7. Cook for 20 minutes uncovered and without stirring *then* stir well, and add more stock if necessary. Cook for another 20 minutes until the rice is tender, and garnish with the remaining mussels, prawns and lobster.

8. Serve with a green salad.

Approx. calories per serving: 400

Curried Baked Beans and Drumsticks

Serves 2

2 chicken drumsticks
225 g (8 oz) baked beans
1 teaspoon curry powder
140 ml (¼ pt/½c) chicken stock

1. Remove all skin and fat from the chicken legs, place in a pan with the stock, cover and simmer gently for 15 minutes. Remove the chicken from the stock and grill until crisp.

2. While these are grilling pour the baked beans into a pan, sprinkle with curry powder and heat through.

3. Serve with the grilled chicken and a foil baked jacket potato or wholemeal rolls and a lettuce and tomato salad with a sweet vinegar dressing.

Approx. calories per serving: 250

Gardener's Baked Beans

Serves 4–6

140 ml (¼ pt/½c) chicken stock
½ small cauliflower, broken into small florets
1 finely chopped onion
25 g (1 oz) canned sweetcorn kernels

25 g (1 oz) French beans, chopped into 25 mm/1" length
25 g (1 oz) fresh or frozen peas
225 g (8 oz) baked beans

1. Heat through all chopped vegetables in the chicken stock for 5 minutes. Strain and heat with the baked beans in a pan for 10 minutes. Season to taste.
2. Garnish with watercress and serve with wholemeal toast.

Approx. calories per serving: 75

Baked Beans on Toast

Serves 1

1 slice wholemeal bread
1 teaspoon tomato puree
225 g (8 oz) baked beans

1. Toast the bread, spread with tomato puree and top with the baked beans.

Approx. calories per serving: 280

Spinach Cream

Serves 2

200 g (8 oz) chopped spinach
200 g (8 oz) mashed, boiled potatoes
100 g (4 oz/½c) curd cheese
100 g (4 oz) canned sweetcorn
Low sodium salt and pepper
Mixed herbs

1. Boil the potatoes and mash them, add salt and pepper to taste. Steam the chopped spinach quickly to soften it, combine it with the mashed potatoes, stir in the curd cheese and sweetcorn. Serve while hot on wholemeal toast and sprinkle with mixed herbs. (This makes a filling snack lunch.)

Approx. calories per serving: 240

Haddock with Dill

Serves 4

570 g (1¼ lb) haddock fillets
skimmed milk
1 teaspoon dill weed (chopped)
Low sodium salt — salt substitute
Pepper
1 level tablespoon low-fat spread
1–2 level tablespoons wholemeal flour
1 hard-boiled egg
340 g (12 oz) cooked green beans

1. Divide the haddock into 4 portions, place in a saucepan, add the dill, low sodium salt and pepper and cover with the milk. Simmer gently for 8–10 minutes. Drain, but keep the liquid and keep the fish hot.
2. Melt the low-fat spread in a saucepan, stir in the flour and add the liquid from the fish, stirring constantly until it thickens. Season to taste.
3. Chop the egg and stir into the sauce. Serve over the fish with green beans.

Approx. calories per serving: 243

Prawn Plaice Rolls

Serves 4

4 115 g (4 oz) plaice fillets
170 g (6 oz) prawns
225 g (8 oz) cooked brown rice (weighed when uncooked)
1 level tablespoon low-fat spread
Pinch of turmeric or affron
Pinch of paprika
Low sodium salt — salt substitute
Pepper
Cucumber strips for garnish

Prawn sauce

For the prawn sauce, place all ingredients into a saucepan and stir continually over a low heat until the sauce thickens. Put aside and pour over plaice rolls before serving.

2 level teaspoons wholemeal flour
280 ml (½ pt/1c) skimmed milk
60 g (2 oz) prawns
3 tablespoons natural yoghurt
1 tablespoon Miso
Low sodium salt — salt substitute
Pepper

1. Lay the fillets out flat and season with low sodium and pepper; add a little lemon juice and tarragon to taste. Divide the prawns among the fillets. Roll up the fillets with the prawns inside and secure with a wooden cocktail stick.
2. Place in an ovenproof dish and dot with low-fat spread. Cover and bake at 190°C/375°F/Gas 5 for 15–20 minutes.

Approx. calories per serving: 231

Trout en Papillote

Serves 2

2 230 g (8 oz) fresh rainbow trout
1 small finely chopped onion
1 level tablespoon dried dill weed
Low sodium salt — salt substitute
Pepper
2 tablespoons dry white wine
1 sliced lemon

1. Wash the trout and dry with a paper towel. Season with low sodium salt and pepper. Open the fish and season inside; stuff with dill, a little onion and a small slice of lemon.
2. Take two pieces of foil and fold each in half to make rectangles 1½ times the length of the fish. Lay each trout on a piece of foil, sprinkle with onion and wine and pleat the foil over the top and sides to enclose it completely. Place the parcels under the grill and cook hot for 10 minutes.
3. Carefully remove the trout from the foil and serve with lemon slices, small jacket-baked potatoes and a mixed lettuce and tomato salad.
4. Alternatively, this dish may be served with small jacket-baked potatoes and boiled broccoli or leeks.

Approx. calories per serving: 350

Mustard Cod

Serves 1

1 170 g (6 oz) cod fillet
1 teaspoon tarragon mustard
1 teaspoon low-fat spread
30 g (1 oz) chopped mushrooms
85 g (3 oz) sliced green beans
1 piece of foil for baking (300 × 200 mm/12 × 8 in)

1. Lay the cod fillet in the centre of the foil. Mix the mustard, low-fat spread and the mushrooms together and spread over the fillet. Fold the foil loosely; place on a baking sheet and bake at 190°C/375°F/Gas 5 for 20–25 minutes.
2. Serve at once with cooked green beans.

Approx. calories per serving: 230

Apple Mackerel

Serves 4

4 230 g (8 oz) fresh mackerel (900 g/2 lb mackerel altogether)
1 medium unpeeled dessert apple, cored and diced
2 sticks chopped celery
85 g (3 oz) finely sliced onion
230 g (8 oz) cooked brown rice
1 teaspoon lemon juice
2 tablespoons skimmed milk
Low sodium salt — salt substitute
Pepper
Cooking foil

1. Remove the fish heads, slit along the belly, gut and wash well. Open the fish and press flat; lift out the backbone. Place the fish on a sheet of foil.
2. Gently sauté the apple, celery and onion in the milk until soft. Stir in the rice and lemon juice, season with low sodium salt and pepper. Use the mixture to stuff the mackerel.
3. Completely enclose the stuffed fish in foil and grill for 15–20 minutes. Alternatively, the dish may be baked in the oven at 190°C/375°F/Gas 5 for 30 minutes.

4. The skin should be removed before eating the fish.
5. This dish goes well with jacket-baked potatoes and coleslaw.

Approx. calories per serving: 325

Curried Fish Risotto

Serves 6

570 g (1¼ lb) rock or monk fish
170 g (6 oz) brown rice
230 g (8 oz) coarsely chopped onion
170 g (6 oz) sliced green peppers
1–2 level tablespoons sultanas (optional)
510 g (18 oz) cooked red kidney beans
1 heaped tsp Vecon in 140 ml (¼ pt/½c) hot water
Spring onions for garnish

Curry Sauce

300 ml (½ pt/ 1c) skimmed milk
2 level tablespoons wholemeal flour
1 level teaspoon pulverised sunflower seeds
2–3 teaspoons curry power to taste
2 tablespoons Miso

1. Remove the bones from the fish, cut in cubes and set aside.
2. Cook the rice in boiling salted water for about 25 minutes.
3. Meanwhile simmer the onion in the Vecon until soft and add the sliced peppers and sultanas.
4. Prepare the curry sauce by placing all the ingredients in a saucepan and bring to the boil, stirring constantly until it thickens.
5. Add the sauce to the onion and peppers and then add the fish . . . cover the pan and simmer gently for 15 minutes to cook the fish. Carefully fold in the rice and serve in a deep dish with a side dish of red kidney beans garnished with spring onions.
6. Serve hot or cold.

Approx. calories per serving: 338

BAKED POTATOES

With an imaginative filling, jacket potatoes make a delicious meal all on their own, served with some salad.

Approx. calories per serving: 150

Tofu and Spinach Filling

Serves 4

225 g (8 oz) fresh spinach
1 sliced onion
100 g (4 oz) Tofu
2 chopped tomatoes
25 g (1 oz) sesame seeds
57 ml (2 fl oz / ¼ c) yoghurt or cottage cheese (optional)
25 g (1 oz) chopped roast almonds (optional)
Low sodium salt — salt substitute
Pepper
Bicarbonate of soda

1. Wash the spinach and put it wet into a pan with a sprinkling of low sodium salt and bicarbonate of soda and steam over a high heat for about 15 minutes until tender. Drain, chop finely and set aside.
2. Gently heat the sliced onion in a pan for 5 minutes with 4 tablespoons stock. Drain the Tofu, add it to the pan and mash with the onion. Continue cooking for 5 minutes.
3. Add tomatoes, spinach, sesame seeds, low sodium salt and pepper to taste. Mix thoroughly, add yoghurt or cottage cheese and sliced roast almonds to taste.

4. Scoop out a little flesh from each potato, mash with the filling, heat through and replace in the potatoes.
5. Sufficient for about 4 potatoes.

Approx. calories per serving: 173

Mushroom and Olive Filling

Serves 4

100 g (4 oz) mushrooms
12 stuffed olives
57 ml (2 fl oz/¼c) plain yoghurt
Low sodium salt — salt substitute
Pepper
3 tablespoons chicken stock

1. Clean and chop the mushrooms and simmer gently in a pan in 3 tbsp chicken stock until just tender. Slice the olives, mix into the mushrooms and season with low sodium salt and pepper. Cut slits into the cooked potatoes and divide the filling evenly. Spoon over yoghurt.
2. Sufficient for about four potatoes.

Approx. calories per serving: 110

Kidney Bean and Tomato Filling

Serves 4

1 onion
1 green pepper
1 stick celery
57 ml (2 fl oz/¼c) plain yoghurt
4 medium tomatoes
275 g (10 oz) cooked kidney beans
1–2 teaspoons chilli powder to taste
Low sodium salt — salt substitute
Pepper

1. Put the chopped onion, green pepper and celery into a pan, with 2

tablespoons low sodium salted water. Cover and heat gently under tender.
2. Add the diced tomatoes, beans, chilli powder and low sodium salt and pepper to taste. Add a little water and simmer for 30 minutes until reduced to a fairly thick sauce. Stir in the yoghurt to taste and heat gently. Divide the sauce over split potatoes. Sufficient for about 4 potatoes.

Approx. calories per serving: 200

Onion and Bacon Filling

Serves 2

2 sliced onions
2–4 tablespoons beef stock
2 tablespoons soya bacon pieces (hydrated)
½ crushed garlic clove (optional)
2 teaspoons chopped fresh basil

1. In a pan, heat the onion and garlic in a little beef stock with the bacon for 5 minutes and season with low sodium salt and pepper.
2. Add the basil with a little more stock, if desired. Heat well through and divide the topping over the split potatoes.

Approx. calories per serving: 160

SALADS AND SALAD DRESSINGS

Broccoli and Egg Salad

Serves 2

450 g (1 lb) broccoli (broken into sprigs)
6 spring onions (chopped)
2 tablespoons plain yoghurt
2 tablespoons cottage cheese
2 hard boiled eggs (sliced) egg yolks removed if desired
Low sodium salt and pepper
A sprinkling of paprika
½ dessert apple (sliced)

1. Cook broccoli sprigs in a little salted boiling water for about 10 minutes (until just tender).
2. Put broccoli in a bowl with sliced egg, apple and spring onions. Mix cottage cheese and yoghurt with salt and pepper, spoon over salad and top with sliced eggs. Sprinkle with paprika.

Approx. calories per serving: 205

Egg and Shrimp Salad

Serves 1

1 hard boiled egg (chopped)
100 g (4 oz) prawns/shrimps
75 g (3 oz/½c) coleslaw (in oil free French dressing)
1 heaped tablespoon cottage cheese
½ box cress (chopped)

1. Serve on a bed of Webbs (if available) or normal lettuce.

2. Mix prawns, coleslaw and cress, spoon onto lettuce. Arrange egg pieces on the salad and top with cottage cheese.
3. Season with paprika, salt and pepper and lemon juice.

Approx. calories per serving: 205

Shrimp and Root Salad

Serves 1

125 g (5 oz) shrimps/prawns
85 g (3 oz) cooked beetroot (diced)
2 medium carrots (shredded)
2 tablespoons cottage cheese
½ small lettuce (shredded)

Dressing

Juice of 1 lemon
2 tablespoons vinegar
1 tablespoon water
2 tablespoons plain low fat yoghurt
3–4 drops sweetener (about 1 tablet)
Low sodium salt and pepper
2 tablespoons chopped fresh chives

1. Prepare dressing and pour over beetroot, carrots and cottage cheese — toss. Arrange shrimps on a bed of lettuce and then top with mixed salad.

Approx. calories per serving: 230

Vegetable Salad

Serves 2

½ medium cauliflower (florets)
2 sticks broccoli (sliced)
2 large leeks (thickly sliced)
2 large plums (chopped)

½ green pepper (cubed)
1 heaped tablespoon cottage cheese

1. Blanch the vegetables by boiling in salted water for about 5 minutes. Drain and leave to cool.
2. When cool, mix with chopped plums and pepper, top with cottage cheese and season with low sodium salt and pepper.

Approx. calories per serving: 82

Kidney Bean Salad

Serves 6

115 g (4 oz) dried kidney beans (soaked overnight) or
425 g (15 oz) red kidney beans
115 g (4 oz) frozen French beans
1 cauliflower, broken into florets
1 small onion, peeled and chopped
115 g (4 oz/½c) cottage cheese
The juice of 1 lemon
4 tablespoons mustard French dressing
Low sodium salt

1. Drain the beans, place in a saucepan and cover with water. Bring to the boil, add a little low sodium salt, cover and simmer for about 1 hour until tender. Drain and rinse in cold water.
2. Cook the French beans in boiling salted water for 2 minutes and drain. Mix the kidney beans, cauliflower, French beans, onion and cottage cheese in a salad bowl. Mix the lemon juice and dressing together, pour over the salad and toss well. Leave to stand for 30 minutes.

Approx. calories per serving: 210

Hot Cabbage Salad

Serves 2

½ shredded white cabbage
3 finely sliced carrots

1 or 2 tablespoons raisins
1 small shredded apple
1 teaspoon fresh marjoram or ½ teaspoons dried marjoram
About 10 drops liquid sweetener
Low sodium salt
Pepper
140 ml (5 fl oz/ ¾c) natural yoghurt

1. Place the vegetables, apple and raisins in a large pan with about 3 tablespoons of water and heat for 3–4 minutes stirring continually. Mix the herbs, sweetener, low sodium salt and pepper to taste into the yoghurt and stir into the vegetables. Heat through very gently and serve at once.

Approx. calories per serving: 150

Nutty Ham Coleslaw

Serves 2

75 g (3 oz/ ½c) coleslaw in oil-free French dressing
50 g (2 oz) ham (lean and diced) or ham flavoured soya chunks (hydrated)
1 stick celery (sliced)
2 medium tomatoes (sliced)
1 large carrot (shredded)
12 g (½ oz) sultanas
12 g (½ oz) salted peanuts

Dressing

3 tablespoons low fat yoghurt
1 flat teaspoon mild English mustard
2-3 drops sweetener
1 tablespoon vinegar
1 tablespoon water
Low sodium salt and pepper to taste
1 small clove garlic (crushed)
½ small onion (finely chopped) if desired

1. Mix all ingredients, prepare salad dressing, pour over salad and toss.

Approx. calories per serving: 228

Red Cabbage Slaw

Serves 6

1 large red cabbage (shredded)
1 small white cabbage (shredded)
2 dessert apples (sliced)
140 ml (5 fl oz / ¾c) plain yoghurt
1 tablespoon vinegar
1–1½ tablets sweetener
Salt and pepper
75 g (3 oz) walnut halves

1. Mix the cabbage with the apple in a bowl. Combine the yoghurt, vinegar, sweetener and salt and pepper to taste and mix well with the slaw.
2. Chill for at least an hour and serve topped with nuts.

Approx. calories per serving: 160

Curried Apple Coleslaw

Serves 2

½ small white cabbage (grated)
2 carrots (grated)
½ small onion (grated)
2 dessert apples (chopped)
25–50 g (1–2 oz) sultanas
2 teaspoons curry powder
6 tablespoons plain yoghurt
Squeeze of lemon
5–10 drops sweetener (optional)

1. Put prepared cabbage, carrots, onion and apples in a bowl with the sultanas and mix well.
2. Stir curry powder and lemon juice into the yoghurt and pour over salad.

Approx. calories per serving: 160

Chicken Curry Salad

Serves 1

1 small apple (cored, thinly sliced)
125 g (5 oz) roast chicken meat (skin and fat removed) cubed
1 stick celery (sliced)
1 bunch watercress (chopped)
1 large tomato (halved and sliced)
½ small onion (finely chopped)

Curry Sauce

2 tablespoons low fat plain yoghurt
1 flat tablespoon cottage cheese
2 tablespoons vinegar
5–8 drops artificial sweetener
1 tablespoon water
Low sodium salt, pepper and curry powder (mild) to taste

1. Mix all prepared ingredients and toss with curry dressing.
2. Serve on a bed of tender lettuce leaves. (All salads can be served with additional lettuce, sliced cucumber or watercress if desired.)

Approx. calories per serving: 300

Spinach Salad

Serves 2

225 g (8 oz) fresh young spinach
3 tomatoes (sliced)
3 stick celery (sliced)
10 black olives (chopped — stones removed)
75 g (3 oz) hazelnuts/pine nuts

1. Wash, drain and chop spinach.
2. Toss all vegetables with mustard dressing and sprinkle with nuts and olives.

Approx. calories per serving: 285

Fennel Salad

Serves 2

1 large grapefruit
1 large fennel
1 cucumber (chunked)
6 radishes (sliced)
1 head chicory (sliced)
1 tablespoon chopped fresh mint
140 ml (5 fl oz/¾c) plain natural yoghurt*
Salt and pepper

1. Finely grate the grapefruit peel and reserve on one side. Peel and divide the grapefruit into segments.
2. Remove base and coarse outer leaves from fennel and slice inside finely. Combine all washed prepared ingredients (grapefruit, fennel, cucumber, radishes and chicory) in a bowl.
3. Mix the mint into the yoghurt, season with salt and pepper and pour over the salad — sprinkle with a little grapefruit peel.

*A few drops artificial sweetener can be added to the yoghurt to round off the taste.

Approx. calories per serving: 100

Creamy Cucumber

Serves 2

4 tablespoons cottage cheese
A little milk
½–1 teaspoon ground cumin
Low sodium salt and pepper
3 tomatoes (sliced)
1 large cucumber (sliced)
Watercress to garnish

1. Rub cottage cheese through a sieve and mix with a little milk to achieve a creamy consistency. Season with cumin, salt and pepper.
2. mix sliced cucumber into cheese dressing, stand for 10 minutes and serve topped with tomatoes and watercress.

Approx. calories per serving: 100

Chinese Leaves and Avocado Salad

Serves 4

1 small head Chinese leaves (chopped)
1 small green pepper (chopped)
2 sticks celery (chopped)
½ small red cabbage (chopped)
2 tomatoes (sliced)
1 large avocado (sliced)
50 g (2 oz) raisins
50 g (2 oz) toasted flaked almonds
Lemon vinegar dressing.

1. Mix all prepared ingredients in a bowl with raisins and the lemon vinegar dressing. Sprinkle nuts over the top.

Approx. calories per serving: 250

Cucumber Dill Salad

Serves 2

1 large cucumber
3 tablespoons fresh chopped dill
140 ml (5 fl oz/¾ c) plain yoghurt (1 carton)
1–2 tablespoons vinegar
5–10 drops sweetener
Low sodium salt and pepper and paprika

1. Mix yoghurt with vinegar, dill, sweetener, salt, pepper and paprika to taste and mix with cucumber.
2. Serve garnished with a sprinkling of paprika.

Approx. calories per serving: 60

Mixed Crunchy Salad

Serves 2

¼ cucumber (sliced)
1 small apple (quartered and sliced)
2 large plums (sliced)
2 medium carrots (sliced thinly)
1 large tomato (sliced)
½ medium onion (finely chopped)
1 heaped tablespoon cottage cheese

1. Serve on a bed of chopped lettuce.
2. Mix all ingredients, toss in a sweet vinegar dressing and spoon onto the bed of lettuce. Top with cottage cheese (and if available, chopped cress and chives).

Approx. calories per serving: 80

Mixed Salad

Serves 4–6

1 small Webbs lettuce (chopped)
1 small soft lettuce (chopped)
4 sticks celery (sliced)
4 tomatoes (sliced)
4 small courgettes (sliced)
8 radishes (sliced)
50 g (2 oz) button mushrooms (sliced)
Chopped fresh parsley
¼ small cauliflower (broken into florets and blanched for 1 minute)

1. Serve with sweet vinegar dressing (page 102).
2. Arrange the two lettuces on a serving dish. In a bowl mix the sliced celery, tomatoes, courgettes and radishes with dressing and pile onto lettuce. Top with cauliflower, mushrooms and parsley.

Approx. calories per serving: 25

Apple Lettuce

Serves 4

2 small dessert apples (thinly sliced)
1 large lettuce (or 1 small normal and 1 small Webbs)
1 cucumber (sliced)
2 slices well toasted wholemeal bread, cubed
Fresh chopped chives

1. Mix shredded lettuce, the sliced cucumber and apple with the wholemeal cubes and top with yoghurt vinegar dressing (page 100) and chives.

Approx. calories per serving: 70

Winter Salad

Serves 2

½ small head Chinese leaves (chopped)
2 sticks celery (chopped)
100 g (4 oz) Brussel sprouts (grated)
1 large dessert pear (diced)
100 g (4 oz) parsnips (grated)
Salt and pepper
2 tomatoes (sliced)
¼ curly endive (chicory)

1. Toss all prepared ingredients except chicory and tomatoes in a bowl with mustard dressing and heap onto a bed of chicory on a serving platter.
2. Garnish with tomatoes.

Approx. calories per serving: 100

Crunchy Cauliflower Salad

Serves 2

100 g (4 oz) soya beans, soaked in water overnight
1 small cauliflower (broken into florets)

1–2 sticks celery (sliced)
1 small cucumber (sliced)
1–2 carrots (thinly sliced)
50 g (2 oz) dried apricots, soaked in water overnight
(coarsely chopped)
4–6 tablespoons yoghurt or green goddess dressing

1. Drop the soya beans in a pot of hot water, bring to the boil; lower the heat and simmer for 45 minutes. Drain and cool.
2. Blanch cauliflower florets for 5 minutes in boiling salted water, drain and mix in a bowl with celery, cucumber, carrots and apricots. Pour in the dressing and top with soya beans.

Approx. calories per serving: 300

California Salad

Serves 2

1 large peach (sliced)
2 sticks celery (chopped)
50 g (2 oz) mushrooms (finely sliced)
½ cucumber (sliced)
1 small red pepper (diced)
2 tomatoes (quartered)
1 large orange (segmented and sliced)
1 large banana (sliced)
½ lettuce (chopped)
225 g (8 oz/1c) cottage cheese
Watercress to garnish
140 ml (¼ pt/½c) lemon dressing

1. Arrange lettuce on a serving plate. Mix all other fruit and vegetables, pour salad dressing over and toss.
2. Then pile salad onto lettuce and top with cottage cheese and watercress.

Approx. calories per serving: 220

Lemon Dressing

3 tablespoons lemon juice
2 tablespoons water
1 tablespoon vingar
About 10 drops (1 tablet) sweetener
Low sodium salt and pepper

1. Simply whisk all ingredients and season to taste. Store in refrigerator.

Approx. calories per serving: 20

Sensible Vinaigrette

3 tablespoons wine vinegar
½–1 teaspoon mustard (French/English)
1 tablespoon skimmed milk
2 teaspoons chopped fresh herbs
Low sodium salt and pepper

1. Thoroughly whisk all ingredients, starting with the mustard and a little vinegar.
2. Store in refrigerator.

Approx. calories per serving: 30

Yoghurt Vinaigrette

3 tablespoons wine vinegar
1 teaspoon mustard
3 tablespoons plain yoghurt
2 teaspoons chopped fresh herbs
½ tablet sweetener (optional)
Low sodium salt and pepper

1. Prepare as for the sensible vinaigrette.

Approx. calories per serving: 60

Coconut Dressing

50 g (2 oz/¼c) cottage cheese
50 g (2 oz/¼c) skimmed milk cottage cheese
1 tablespoon dessicated coconut
1 tablespoon milk
1–2 tablets sweetener (dissolved in some milk)

1. If using tablets gently warm milk and dissolve.
2. Pass cottage cheese through a sieve and mash with other ingredients until smooth and creamy.

Approx. calories per serving: 230

Italian Dressing

4 tablespoons vinegar
1 tablespoon yoghurt
½ tablet sweetener
1 clove garlic (crushed)
¼ onion (cut and mashed up)
1 teaspoon chopped fresh basil (½ teaspoon dried)

1. Whisk all ingredients with crushed onion and garlic, season to taste and leave to stand briefly in order to let the flavours mingle.

Approx. calories per serving: 35

Sensible 1,000 Island Dressing

300 ml (½ pt/1½c) yoghurt
2 tablespoons cottage cheese
1 tablespoon tomato puree
1 finely chopped hard boiled egg — white only
(5 chopped stuffed olives — optional)
*20 drops/2 tablets sweetener
Low sodium salt and pepper

1. Pass cottage cheese through a sieve.
2. Mix all ingredients very thoroughly, taste, and adjust sweetening.

*Tablets dissolved in a teaspoon hot water.

Approx. calories per serving: 180
including olives: 300

Sweet Vinegar Dressing

(Viennese Dressing)

4 tablespoons tarragon vinegar (though ordinary vinegar is acceptable)
1 tablespoon water
1 tablet sweetener
Low sodium salt and pepper
2 tablespoons plain yoghurt (optional)

Approx. calories per serving: 40

DESSERTS

Summer Fruit Salad

Serves 8

1 grapefruit
1 orange
1 dessert apple (Golden Delicious)
1 crisp green apple
100 g (4 oz) strawberries
1 small pineapple
1 cucumber
1 pear
1 thick slice honey melon (or sugar)
100 g (4 oz) raspberries

1. Prepare and cut all fruit and mix with juice of ½ lemon and 6–8 tablets sweetener.
2. Serve with sweet yoghurt cream.

Approx. calories per serving: 47

Fresh Fruit Trifle

Serves 10

3 ripe bananas
4 dessert apples
50 g (2 oz) sultanas
1 chopped pineapple
450 g (1 lb) plums or any soft fruit
300 ml (10 fl oz/1½c) natural low fat yoghurt

2 tablespoons fruit bran
2 drops vanilla essence
10 drops artificial sweetener
1 tablespoon sunflower seeds

1. Mash the bananas, grate the apples and mix together.
2. Mix the yoghurt, vanilla essence and sweetener to taste. Layer in a trifle bowl the pineapple pieces, chopped plums, mashed bananas, apples and a layer of fruit bran. Top with the yoghurt and sprinkle a little bran and sunflower seeds on top.
3. Place in the fridge for ½ an hour before serving.

Approx. calories per serving: 100

Summer Pudding

Serves 6

200 g (½ lb) *strawberries*
200 g (½ lb) *raspberries*
200 g (½ lb) *blackberries*
200 g (½ lb) *blackcurrants*
200 g (½ lb) *redcurrants*

1. Clean and prepare all fruit and put it into a large pot, cook over a gentle heat for 15 minutes.
2. Meanwhile, line a bowl with cling plastic, letting it hang over the edges, and line this with tightly packed wholemeal bread slices (crusts removed) — 5 should do.
3. When fruit is cooked, sweeten to taste with sweetener and drain — keeping juice in a jar in the fridge as flavouring for yoghurt. Simply pack the cooked fruit onto the wholemeal bread slices, press down with a flat spoon and cover the top with more bread. Chill overnight in the fridge, weighed down with a plate and some weights. Before serving, simply tip onto a plate using the cling film.
4. Serve with sweet yoghurt cream, and — if desired — the fruit juice.

Approx. calories per serving: 50

Banana Bake

Serves 3–4

4 large bananas
25 g (1 oz) raisins
75 g (3 oz/1⅓c) cottage cheese
100 g (4 oz) wholemeal flour
Artificial sweetener — to taste

1. Slice the bananas and place them in a dish, sprinkle on the raisins. Rub the cottage cheese into the wholemeal flour and add the sweetener to taste. Sprinkle over sliced bananas. Bake in the oven until brown, approx. 20 minutes at 180°C/350°F/Gas 4. Serve with yoghurt cream.

Approx. calories per serving: 195

Strawberry Whip

Serves 4

450 g (1 lb) strawberries
2 egg whites
Lemon juice
Liquid sweetener
2 heaped tablespoons low-fat yoghurt

1. Mash the strawberries, add yoghurt, sweetener and lemon juice to taste. This mixture can stay in the fridge for hours if desired.
2. Not more than ½ hour before serving, beat egg whites and fold into the mixture. Serve immediately, garnished with strawberries.

Strawberry Sorbet

1. Freeze exactly the same strawberry mixture without egg whites, beaten up twice before completely frozen (at ½ hour intervals).
2. Before serving, mix with beaten egg whites.

Approx. calories per serving: 40

Strawberry Soufflé

Serves 4

450 g (1 lb) strawberries
4 egg whites (large eggs)
8–10 tablets sweetener (crushed and pulverised)
Squeeze of lemon

1. Press cleaned strawberries through a sieve or blend in a liquidizer to a thick puree. Mix well with sweetener and a drop of lemon juice.
2. Whisk the egg whites until stiff enough to hold firm peaks, and gently fold into strawberry puree.
3. Pour into a lightly greased souffle dish and bake for about 30 minutes until well risen — 180°C/350°F/Gas 4.
4. Serve at once.

N.B. This soufflé can be made with peaches, apricots, raspberries, blackberries, cherries (no stones), plums, gooseberries, bananas and almost any ripe reasonably soft fruit.

The raw soufflé mixture makes a perfect pudding *uncooked* with a little extra chopped fruit and served with a yoghurt cream. (Plain yoghurt mixed with sweetener.)

Approx. calories per serving: 40

Spicy Baked Pears

Serves 2–3

4 large pears
'Pear'n'Apple' spread (concentrated pear and apple juice)
Mixed spice

1. Cut the pears in half and remove the core. Lay the pears in a dish and sprinkle with mixed spice. Spread one teaspoon of spread on each pear half, cover with foil and bake for 20 minutes — 180°C/350°F/Gas 4.
2. Serve with yoghurt cream.

Approx. calories per serving: 94

Banana Whip

Serves 2–3

140 ml (5 fl oz/1 ¼c) natural yoghurt
2 ripe bananas
25 g (1 oz) chopped dates
25 g (1 oz) chopped walnuts
Cinnamon
Artificial sweetener
2 tablespoons bran plus (fine bran)

1. Mash the bananas with the sweetener, mix in the yoghurt, cinnamon and dates. Place in a dessert glass and sprinkle with walnuts.

N.B. This dessert can also be made in the blender and is a good way to get unprocessed bran into your diet.

Approx. calories per serving: 150

Hot Stuffed Peaches

Serves 4

4 large firm peaches
75 g (3 oz/½c) dried wholemeal breadcrumbs
50 g (2 oz/¼c) cottage cheese
4 large prunes (soaked in water overnight)
25 g (1 oz) flaked almonds
5–6 tablets sweetex (to taste)

1. Wash and halve the peaches, scoop out some of the flesh with a teaspoon leaving a firm bowl. Chop the flesh, and mix it in a bowl with the breadcrumbs. Mash the cottage cheese (pass through a sieve) drain and finely chop the prunes — removing stones — mix them with the cottage cheese and beat with the peach flesh and breadcrumbs, adding crushed or liquid sweetener to taste. Fill into the peaches and sprinkle with flaked almonds.
2. Heat through under a gentle grill for about 5 minutes.
3. Serve with yoghurt cream (plain yoghurt mixed with sweetener).

Approx. calories per serving: 133

Fruit Mince Crumble

Serves 4

50 g (2 oz) sultanas
50 g (2 oz) raisins
50 g (2 oz) currants
1 dessert apple (grated)
Rind of 1 orange
4 tablespoons 'Whole Earth' Hedgerow jam (no added sugar)
Mixed spice (approx 1 teaspoon)

Crumble

75 g (3 oz/⅓c) cottage cheese
100 g (4 oz) wholemeal flour or oats
Artificial sweetener to taste
Chopped nuts

1. Mix the dried fruit, grated apple, orange rind, jam and mixed spice and place in a dish.
2. Rub the cottage cheese into the flour and add a few drops of artificial sweetener if required. Sprinkle the crumble mixture onto the fruit and top with chopped nuts. Cook in a moderate oven for 20 minutes — until brown. Serve with yoghurt cream.

Approx. calories per serving: 147

Crunchy Bran

This crunchy bran recipe is simply a method of making the dry, flaky bran we eat every day more appetising, and in this form can be enjoyed as a cereal all on its own.

375 g (13.2 oz) bran
200 ml (⅓ pt/¾c) warm water
180 g (6 oz) 'whole earth jam' (use whichever flavour you prefer)

1. Dissolve the jam in the warm water in a large bowl.
2. Pour bran over liquid and mix very thoroughly so that the bran is well moistened through. Spread mixture evenly on a baking tray, and bake at a low heat for 1 hour. Keep crunchy bran in tins, plastic containers or plastic bags; it keeps very well and can be eaten just like ordinary bran.

Approx. calories per serving: 20

Fruity Bread Pudding

Serves 6–8

200 g (8 oz/1⅓c) *fine wholemeal breadcrumbs*
100 g (4 oz) *mixed dried fruit*
1 *egg white*
2 *tablespoons 'Whole Earth' jam (Hedgerow or Blackberry)*
1 *teaspoon mixed spice*
Little skimmed milk

1. Place the breadcrumbs in a bowl with the dried fruit. Add the egg white, whole earth jam and spice and enough skimmed milk to make the mixture totally moist. Leave this to stand for 15 minutes to soak; then press into a dish and bake for 20 minutes until brown. 180°C/350°F/Gas 4.
2. This can be served hot with yoghurt or yoghurt cream or it can be eaten cold in thin slices.

Approx. calories per serving: 100

Deep Dish Plum Pie

Serves 4–6

75 g (3 oz/⅓c) *skimmed milk cottage cheese*
175 g (6 oz) *plain wholemeal flour*
2–3 *tablespoons cold water*
Pinch salt
4 *tablets sweetex*

Filling

675 g (1½ lb) *plum*
10–15 *tablets artificial sweetener (crushed)*
1–2 *teaspoons cinnamon (optional)*
Squeeze of lemon
1 *tablespoon water*

1. Rub the cottage cheese into the flour and add the salt and sweetener. Add enough water to hold dough together and knead briefly. Chill in fridge for 30 minutes.
2. Then roll out flour into a round 1 in bigger all round than the pie dish — leave on side.

3. Wash, halve and stone plums, and in a bowl mix with sweetener, cinnamon and lemon. Pile into dish and cover plums with pastry, pressing edges onto pie dish (use a little water).

4. Brush pie top with water and bake in the preheated oven — 200°C/400°F/Gas 6 — for 20 minutes before turning down to 180°C/350°F/Gas 4 for 20 more minutes.

5. Serve with sweet yoghurt cream.

Approx. calories per serving: 128

Apricot Sponge Flan

Serves 4

Sponge base

85 g (3 oz) wholemeal flour
3 egg whites
3 tablespoons plain low fat yoghurt
About 8 tablets sweetener (to taste)
2 teaspoons baking powder
Vanilla essence

Filling

450 g (1 lb) apricots (ripe) halved
mixed with a little artificial sweetener if desired
100 g (4 oz) fruit bran sprinkled on top

1. Thinly grease a flat biscuit tray. Whisk together the egg whites, yoghurt, vanilla and sweetener for about 10–15 minutes. Sift together wholemeal flour and baking powder and lightly fold into whisked mixture. Pour base onto tray and cover evenly with apricot halves. Sprinkle with fruit bran and bake at a medium heat for 15–20 minutes. When cold cut into squares.

2. Serve with yoghurt cream.

Approx. calories per serving: 115

Apricot Rice

Serves 2

100 g (4 oz) short grain, brown, unpolished rice
250 ml (½ pt/1c) skimmed milk
Liquid artificial sweetener
Whole earth apricot jam (no added sugar)

1. Boil the rice in water for 20 minutes until it is nearly cooked. Then wash the rice in boiling water to get rid of the excess starch. Place in a saucepan with the skimmed milk and sweetener to taste, simmer until the milk is absorbed by the rice. Place in a dish with the apricot jam spread on top, heat through in a low oven for 10 minutes and serve with a spoonful of natural low fat yoghurt.

Approx. calories per serving: 263

Apple and Raisin Pie

Serves 4

Base

75 g (3 oz) wholemeal flour (fine ground)
25 g (1 oz) soya flour
50 g (2 oz) curd cheese
Cold water
Pinch of salt

1. Make the case as you would for the golden carrot quiche. Line a lightly greased pie dish.

Filling

3 cooking apples (medium)
75 g (3 oz) raisins
75 g (3 oz) fine oats
75 g (3 oz/⅓c) cottage cheese
Mixed spice
Sweetener

1. Slice the apples and lay inside the pie case. Sprinkle with the raisins and

artificial sweetener (if required). Rub the cottage cheese into the oats with some sweetener and spice (approx ½ teaspoon). Sprinkle the crumb mixture on top and bake for 25 minutes until brown, at 180°C/350°F/Gas 4.

2. Serve with yoghurt cream.

The same base can be filled with any 'Whole Earth' jam to make a 'sugar free' jam tart.

Approx. calories per serving: 160

Blackberry Cheesecake

Serves 6

8–10 tablets sweetener (pulverised or liquid)
3 egg whites (whipped)
300 g (11 oz/1¼c) cottage cheese
300 g (11 oz/1¼c) curd cheese
Grated rind of 1 lemon

Pastry

100 g (4 oz) wholemeal flour
25 g (1 oz/⅛c) cottage cheese
4–6 tablespoons skimmed milk
2 tablets sweetener (pulverised or liquid)
Pinch salt
4 slices wholewheat crispbread (crumbled into flour)

1. Pass the 25 g cottage cheese through a sieve and mix with a little milk. Mix flour with finely crumbled crispbread, a pinch of salt and the sweetener, and then cream with cottage cheese.

2. Press pastry into a slightly greased cake tin and pre-bake for 15 minutes. Meanwhile, pass the 300 g cottage cheese through a sieve, and then mix well with curd cheese, lemon rind and sweetener. Gently fold in lightly beaten egg whites and spoon onto hot (or cooled) pastry. Smooth over top and bake for 20–25 minutes.

3. While cheesecake is in the oven simmer 50 g (2 oz) of whatever fruit desired with sweetener (4 or 5 tablets) for 5–10 minutes. Remove from heat and drain, keeping liquid. Set aside.

4. When cheesecake has set, remove from oven, and while hot, decorate top completely with blackberries (½ strawberries, peach slices or whatever)

and then pour over the warm fruit liquid if desired. Serve with sweet yoghurt cream. Allow to cool a little, and then chill for 1–2 hours in fridge.

Sweet Yoghurt Cream

140 ml (5 fl oz/ ¾c) plain yoghurt
4 tablets sweetener
3–4 drops vanilla essence (optional)

1. Beat well. Keeps well and is delicious almost anywhere where normal fresh cream would be used.

Approx. calories per serving cheesecake 230
cream 90

BISCUITS AND CAKES

Almond Crunchy Biscuits

200 g (8 oz) ground almonds
100 g (4 oz) sesame seeds
3 egg whites
50 g (2 oz) ground rice (brown)
Split almonds
Rice paper
Few drops vanilla essence (6–7 drops)
Artificial sweetener
Little skimmed milk

1. Leave egg whites to stand overnight if possible.
2. Mix all ingredients together and beat well for 10 minutes. Form into a dough and roll out, making into biscuits with a medium biscuit cutter, brush with a little egg white and place a split almond in the centre of each.
3. Bake medium to hot for 20 minutes, turning once.

Approx. calories per biscuit: 70

Macaroons

100 g (4 oz) ground brown rice
100 g (4 oz) ground almonds
25 g (1 oz) soya flour
1 egg white
25 g (1 oz) sesame seed
1 tablespoon yoghurt (natural low fat)
5 tablespoons skimmed milk
Artificial sweetener (as required)
Vanilla essence
Rice paper

114

1. Combine the ground rice, almonds, soya flour and sesame seeds with the egg white, yoghurt and skimmed milk.
2. Stir well with the vanilla essence and artificial sweetener for about 5 minutes. Form the dough into biscuit shapes on the rice paper. Bake for 25 minutes until golden. Split almonds can be sprinkled on the top. 180°C/ 350°F/Gas 4.

Approx. calories per macaroon: 65

Lemon Steamed Sponge

Serves 4

100 g (4 oz) wholemeal flour
2 heaped teaspoons baking powder
2 eggs
Grated rind of 1 lemon
Lemon juice of 1 lemon
3 tablespoons lemon curd
4 tablespoons yoghurt (plain — low fat)
6–7 crushed sweetener tabletrs (or 60–70 drops liquid)

1. Lightly beat the eggs, mix yoghurt with sweetener, lemon rind and lemon juice, and then beat the eggs in a little at a time. Bit by bit sift the flour into the mixture (reserving bran for another recipe) and mix gently.
2. Thinly grease a 900 ml (1½ pt) pudding basin. Spoon in the lemon curd and turn the basin to evenly distribute it over the bottom. Carefully pour in the pudding mixture. Cover the top with a clean kitchen cloth, letting it hang over the sides and secure firmly around edge with string.
3. Stand basin in a steamer and put steamer in a large basin of boiling waer (two-thirds submerged). Steam for at least 1½–2 hours — check from time to time that there is enough water.
4. When ready, tip onto a warmed plate and serve with lemon sauce.

Lemon Sauce

2 lemons
about 150 ml (¼ pt/½c) water
15 g (½ oz) arrowroot
Pinch of grated nutmeg
6–7 tablets sweetener (to taste)

1. Scrape peel off lemons and set aside, then halve and squeeze out all juice. Pour in enough water to make up 300 ml (½ pt/1c) and add the sweetener.
2. Mix the arrowroot with a tablespoon of lemon water to a smooth paste, and heat remainder. When warm, stir arrowroot paste into lemon water, add nutmeg and heat gently until sauce thickens. Transfer sauce to a jug and sprinkle with the lemon peel.

Approx. calories per serving: sponge 160
sauce 70

Christmas Dundee Cake

Serves 10–15

150 g (6 oz) cooking dates
100 g (4 oz) low-fat spread
Grated rind of 1 lemon
3 egg whites
2 tablespoons yoghurt (natural low-fat)
200 g (8 oz) plain wholemeal flour
2 teaspoons baking powder
1 teaspoon mixed spice
450 g (1 lb) mixed, dried fruit
25 g (1 oz) ground almonds
25 g (1 oz) flaked almonds

1. Line a 7–8 inch cake tin with greaseproof paper. Pre-heat oven at 180°C/350°F/Gas 4.
2. Chop the dates and cook in some water in a saucepan until soft. Place the dates, low-fat spread, lemon rind, egg whites and yoghurt into a bowl. Sift in the flour, spice and baking powder — replace the bran left behind in the sieve. Beat vigorously until light and fluffy in texture (can be done in a mixer too!).
3. Stir in the fruit and ground almonds — spoon into the lined tin.
4. Sprinkle with the flaked almonds.
5. Bake for 2½ hours until the cake is risen and golden on top.

75 calories per ounce (normal Christmas Cake with icing and marzipan 330 calories per ounce).

A 'Better' Christmas Pudding

Serves 10–15

200 g (8 oz) cooking dates
140 ml (¼ pt/½c) skimmed milk
200 g (8 oz) low-fat spread (St. Ivel Gold)
2 egg whites
1 tablespoon yoghurt (natural low fat)
1 tablespoon Molasses
1 lemon
100 g (4 oz) chopped raisins
100 g (4 oz) chopped mixed peel
25 g (1 oz) blanched almonds
200 g (8 oz) currants
100 g (4 oz) sultanas
100 g (4 oz) plain wholemeal flour
100 g (4 oz) wholemeal breadcrumbs
½ teaspoon grated nutmeg
½ teaspoon ground ginger
1½ teaspoon mixed spice

1. Chop the dates and cook them in a saucepan with the skimmed milk until they go mushy. Remove from the heat and let them cool. Cream together the low-fat spread and the dates in a big mixing bowl, beat in the egg whites, yoghurt, molasses, lemon rind and juice. Add the other ingredients.
2. Mix well until it becomes a 'dropping' consistency. Fill a lightly greased 2 pint basin or two 1 pint basins.
3. Cover with greaseproof paper and foil and secure with string.
4. Steam for 4 hours topping up with more water if required.
5. Store in a dry place.
6. Steam for another 3 hours before serving.

87 calories per ounce (normal 'shop' pudding 150–200 calories per ounce).

INDEX